101 *ways* to treat your Itch

*From **Roman** times to **Victorian** times,
from **Old Wives Tales** to **Modern Medicine**,
and every **itch** remedy in between.*

HELEN LOCK

First published in 2015 by Helen's Skin Therapy
xmatherapy@gmail.com
www.xmatherapy.com.au
Australia

ISBN: 9780994405555

Subjects: Eczema | Eczema skincare | Psoriasis | Natural treatments
National Library of Australia Dewey Number: 616.51024

Publishing services: Bev Ryan Publishing – www.bevryanpublish.com
Book cover design: Michael Hanrahan Publishing – www.mhpublishing.com.au

Disclaimer
The material in this publication is of the nature of general comment only, and does not
represent professional advice. It is not intended to provide specific guidance for particular
circumstances and it should not be relied on as the basis of any decision to take action or
not take action on any matter which it covers. Readers should obtain professional advice
where appropriate, before making any such decision. To the maximum extent permitted
by law, the author and publisher disclaim all responsibility and liability to any person,
arising directly or indirectly from any person taking or not taking action based on the
information in this publication.

Dedication

This book is dedicated to my sister Wendy, who is an eczema sufferer,
and to my mother, father and family.
It is also in recognition of other 'eczema families' across the world.

Contents

Foreword   vii

Helen's Story   ix

Introduction   xii

A. Acupuncture to Arsenic   15

B. Benzoin to Burdock   26

C. Calendula to Cypress   38

D. Diet   56

E. Echinacea to Evening Primrose Oil   58

F. Fish Oil to Fumitory   69

G. Geranium to Gotu Kola   75

H. Heartsease to Hypnotherapy   83

I. Immunosuppressants to Iron   92

J. Jewelweed to Juniper   94

K. Kukui nut oil to Kunzea   100

L. Lavender to Liquorice   102

M. Magnesium to Myrrh   106

N. Neem   115

O. Oats to Oregon Grape Root   116

P. Parsley to Purslane   120

R. Red Clover to Rosewood   132

S. Safflower Oil to Sweet Orange 140

T. Tamanu Oil to Turmeric 160

V. Vitamins 162

W. Walnut Oil to Witch Hazel 165

Y. Yellow Dock 170

Z. Zinc Oxide 171

Index of Remedies 173

Elektra Magnesium Cream 175

Emma Organics 177

Organic Rosehip Skincare 179

Aviation Hydration Moisturiser 181

XMA Skin Therapy 183

Eczema Association Australasia 185

Foreword

As well as having eczema for most of my life, I have spent almost all of my career working with people with the same skin condition. Most people endeavour to control their itchy skin the best way they can – whether by conventional medicine or by other means.

In my role as President of the Eczema Association of Australasia Inc I talk to a variety of people every day about products that help calm and control the itch associated with eczema. That seems to be the most debilitating aspect of this skin disease – trying to live a productive life and cope with the extreme itchiness all of the time.

Indeed, my own mother used to take a mixture containing camphor oil, which was made up for her by a local pharmacist in order to alleviate her itchy skin. Unfortunately this was to the detriment of her colon, as she now suffers from extremely severe diverticulitis caused by the camphor oil, according to her specialist.

I first met Helen Lock about ten years ago when she visited our office with a skin cream concoction she calls XMA Skin Therapy, which she had whipped up in her kitchen. She was offering it for trial on my 'guinea pigs' who are some loyal members of our Association who offer to trial new products. Helen was looking for feedback on whether her cream worked as well on more people with eczema than just her close family and friends, for whom it had worked amazingly well.

Since that time Helen has been a tireless supporter of our Association, which is the only patient support group for people with eczema in Australia. She has helped out with fundraising and we have often bumped ideas off each other about products and ways of helping people with their skin conditions.

I was delighted when Helen told me she was writing this book and requested my involvement. I wish her lots of luck as a book is a huge undertaking – especially when writing for the first time. I sincerely hope there is something in this book that will help everyone with eczema to relieve their dreaded, persistent and challenging itchy skin.

Cheryl Talent
President
Eczema Association of Australasia Inc
www.eczema.org.au

Helen's Story

My journey into the world of natural skin care products began with my sister Wendy. When Wendy was forced to leave her nursing job due to an acute case of eczema, I decided to take matters into my own hands.

I could see there were already plenty of treatments available on the market, but I didn't know what the long-term effect of any of the chemical ingredients would be. This concerned me. Surely there had to be a more natural and effective alternative?

Armed with nothing more than a bowl and a blender, I took to the kitchen, bathroom and garden in the hopes of finding suitable ingredients. The winning combination became:

- Lavender, sweet orange, shea nut butter, witch hazel, jojoba and grape seed oil from the bathroom cabinet
- Chamomile, sesame oil and olive oil from the kitchen shelf
- Aloe vera plucked from the garden.

With my first concoction ready to go, it was time to put it to the test. I took it to my workplace at the time, a coffee shop at the Royal Brisbane Hospital, and there I handed out sample pots to hospital staff. It was a hit. Soon enough I was spending every weekend making up to 20 pots of the cream for staff.

Despite such quick success, it wasn't until I tuned in to watch a late night martial arts show one evening that I decided to take the cream to the shelves. Three brilliant letters blared at me through the television set that evening: XMA, short for extreme martial arts. Bingo – a light went on in my head. "XMA... xma... eczema!" I immediately trademarked it. To this day people love the name.

I continued making the cream at home for over a year before a move to England prompted me to take it to the next level. News of my impending departure quickly travelled around the hospital. One day one of the nurses came to me and said, "Have a look at my hands." To me they just looked normal; then she said, "My hands have never been this good. What am I going to do if you move to England? How will I get the cream?"

From that moment I knew what I had to do. I told her not to worry.

Nervously, I approached the owner of the hospital pharmacy to ask if he would stock the cream for the staff. To my delight he said yes! The largest hospital in the Southern Hemisphere was about to become the first retail outlet for XMA.

With my first stockist under my belt, I began to research my competition. There was only one other eczema treatment on the market in Australia that used natural ingredients. I was to be the second.

I decided to keep my original ingredients, and added a natural preservative and vitamins A, C and E. Needless to say that was the easy part. Getting the business running over the next few years was an uphill battle filled with lawyers, manufacturers and Therapeutic Goods Administration approval.

Fortunately, today is a different story. Since its beginning in 2002, XMA has become one of the best natural eczema treatment companies in Australia – and the business continues to grow.

From humble beginnings in my kitchen to the development of an additional brand, Aviation Hydration, which is being gifted to celebrities at the Logies, Golden Globes and Oscars, as well as Oprah Winfrey during her 2015 visit to Australia, XMA has grown into a nationwide business, proving that natural medicines can be just as effective – if not more so – than their chemical-filled counterparts.

In this book you will find an historical round-up of recipes and remedies used through the ages*, some no longer recommended today, and many successful ones that use the same natural ingredients found in my moisturisers.

From A to Z, here are 101 ways to treat your itch, naturally.

Helen Lock

---

* *Information on the remedies described in this book is for educational use only and not intended as medical advice. Remedies in this book may trigger side effects and interfere with other medications, herbs and supplements. Please consult your healthcare practitioner (herbalist, naturopath, homeopath or general practitioner) before self-administering a herb or remedy.*

Introduction

First coined in 1933 by Wise and Sulzberger, the term "atopic dermatitis" is used to describe the inherited, chronic skin condition that causes skin to become red, dry, itchy and at times, weepy. More commonly known as eczema, atopic dermatitis usually first appears in early childhood. Some sufferers of eczema may experience symptoms all their lives, while others may experience periods of regression followed by occasional flare-ups. Unfortunately, there is no cure for eczema. The good news however, is that it is manageable, with a number of effective treatments available on the market.

Throughout history, we can see there have been many methods of treating this irritating yet common condition. While there is limited data available on eczema before the Second World War, there is plenty of evidence of skin disease treatments throughout history – some even dating as far back as the 1st century.

Some treatments, like zinc oxide, which is still used in the popular calamine lotion, were a success. Others, like opiates, were phased out, considered useless and even dangerous. Still, topical treatment of the skin is as old as the evolution of man. Instinctively, we try to treat a skin injury or irritation with cooling or soothing substances. Even animals lick their wounds, trusting their instinct and the healing power of saliva.

So when did we take the gigantic leap from folk medicine to modern drug therapy? The question is difficult to answer. The transition from classical to modern scientific medicine is likely to have begun during the Renaissance, between the 15th and 16th centuries. Nevertheless, many centuries would pass before effective topical treatments became widely accepted.

Despite the number of readily available steroid creams on the market today, there is still much that can be learned from ancient medicine and those who used it. One of these people is the Ancient Egyptian pharaoh, Cleopatra, who was renowned not only for her exploits and almost mystical life, but for her beauty and grace. Marcus Tullius Cicero, a Roman philosopher, wrote the following of her: "Her character which pervaded her actions in an inexplicable way when meeting people was utterly spellbinding. The sound of her voice was sweet when she talked."

This extraordinary woman, whom both Caesar and Marc Anthony fell in love with, must have been both beautiful and mesmerizing. And with cleansing creams made of oil and lime, Aleppo soap, Dead Sea salts and donkey milk baths, Cleopatra's beauty regime was legendary in itself. Ancient Egyptians were obsessed with body care, cosmetics, and beauty – and Cleopatra was no exception.

Although there is not enough archaeological evidence to confirm that Cleopatra suffered from a skin ailment, her obsession with bathing in donkey milk and exfoliating with Dead Sea salts to slough off her dry skin raises question marks. To her, beauty was more than skin deep – she wanted to keep her skin blemish free, glowing, and translucent, on display for all to see.

One notable historical figure who did confirm his status as an eczema sufferer was Victorian scientist Charles Darwin. Best known for his work on evolution, this English naturalist and geologist was plagued with a number of ailments for much of his adult life. After repeatedly suffering from an uncommon combination of symptoms that left him severely debilitated for long periods of time, Darwin began recording his symptoms and experiences in a diary. Rashes, itching, fatigue, gastrointestinal problems including pain, nausea, frequent vomiting, a swimming head, severe headaches, trembling, insomnia, joint pain, poor resistance to infections and depression were all part of an extensive list of symptoms noted by the scientist.

In 1849 Darwin tried water therapy at an establishment in Malvern. After just eight days, he experienced a skin eruption all over his legs. Darwin kept records of the effects of the water treatment in his home, and in 1852 discontinued the treatment. Darwin's illness worsened and he began taking arsenic for his many physical and skin ailments. He is believed to have died from chronic arsenic poisoning, possibly caused by the use of arsenic soap to treat his eczema.

Today, many people continue to suffer from this obnoxious itch, with a number of well-known faces reportedly suffering from eczema and psoriasis. But such is the stigma surrounding a skin disease, many celebrities would rather own up to an addiction than admit they have a skin problem.

Let's take a look at 101 ways to treat your itch.

1. Acupuncture

With a history that dates back at least 2000 years ago, acupuncture is one of the oldest and most long-standing health care systems in the world. The ancient Chinese practice involves inserting thin, sterile needles into specific sites of the body, known as acupuncture points. These points are part of a network of invisible channels found throughout the body called meridians. According to practitioners, as long as enough qi (pronounced chee) or 'life energy' flows through the meridians, the body will remain healthy. By inserting needles along the meridians, practitioners work to clear any blockages and encourage the normal flow of qi.

The oldest surviving description is in the Yellow Emperor's Classic of Internal Medicine which was written in China in about 100BC. By the sixth century, the practise of acupuncture had been codified and standardised throughout China, and it remained one of the mainstays of Chinese medicine practice until outlawed in 1929 by the nationalist government of Chiang Kai-shek. The practice of acupuncture continued in rural areas until the ban was lifted by Mao Tse-tung in 1949.

The first information in Europe about acupuncture was published by Dutch traders to Japan in the late eighteenth century. In 1821, the Englishman J.M. Churchill published A Treatise on Acupuncture under the sponsorship of the Royal College of Surgeons and brought knowledge of the practice into the British area of influence.

While skin conditions like eczema manifest externally, acupuncture can be used to treat their root causes, which are often complex and internal, by restoring the balances of internal organs, qi, blood, yin, yang and other energy systems in the body to help nourish and repair skin. Through strengthening the immune system and releasing toxins from the skin, acupuncture is said to decrease the body's sensitivity to external hazards.

Although a number of sessions are usually required, acupuncture can be combined with other anti-itch medicine. Best of all however, this ancient treatment can be used to relieve various itches, as it works from the inside out.

Consult your healthcare practitioner.

2. Almond Oil

AKA: *Prunus amygdalus dulcis*

Popular in both Ancient Greece and Italy, the benefits of almond oil have been well documented throughout history. Light and widely available, sweet almond oil has been used as a moisturiser for centuries. While traditionally cold pressed, much of the almond oil available for sale today is extracted using solvents. This nourishing oil is not only a great emollient, but can also be used to relieve both eczema and itchy scalps.

Scalp Tonic

Massage 1 part rosemary oil with 2 parts almond oil to improve circulation, which may ease itching and help prevent hair follicles for deteriorating.

Consult your healthcare practitioner.

3. Aloe Vera

AKA: *Aloe barbadensis*

Hindu legend has it that the aloe vera plant was first plucked from the Garden of Paradise – and it's not hard to see why. As one of the oldest medicinal plants in history, and a member of the lily family, aloe vera has an almost endless list of uses. A member of the lily family and a favourite among royals and rulers alike, this useful succulent is said to be the reason Alexander the Great conquered the island of Socotra in the Indian Ocean. Following the advice of the great philosopher Aristotle, he seized the island solely for the purpose of obtaining a sufficient supply of the plant to rub on the wounds of his soldiers.

In Ancient Greece aloe vera was used to treat wounds, while in Africa, hunters preferred to rub the plant on their skin to remove their scent before hunting. The mention of aloe vera has even been found in the Egyptian Book of Remedies, with Cleopatra rumoured to have massaged the gel into her skin every day. Napoleon's wife Josephine, on the other hand, supposedly preferred a mixture of milk and aloe to maintain her glowing complexion.

Today the medicinal properties of aloe have been confirmed by science, with research documenting its numerous healing effects. Thanks to its polysaccharides and glycoproteins (carbohydrate molecules and proteins), aloe vera can be used to repair the outer layer of skin in those who suffer from eczema and psoriasis. By cutting open a leaf and applying an aloe vera fillet to the affected area, sufferers of burns, bites and itches will experience almost instant relief. The soothing gel found inside the leaf may also be used as a moisturiser to keep skin smooth and supple due to its ability to improve the skin's oxygen levels and increase the synthesis and strength of both collagen and tissue.

Aloe vera can also be used to help heal wounds without scarring.

Keep an aloe vera plant in a pot by the kitchen windowsill and you will have one of the best skin healing plants on hand.

10 Ways to use Aloe Vera

1. Treat burns and minor cuts
2. Soothe and heal sunburns
3. Take the sting out of insect bites
4. Drink to lower blood sugar levels
5. Drink for digestive purposes
6. Apply to skin infections like boils
7. Take a sip in the morning for a laxative effect
8. Help wounds heal faster
9. Use as a daily moisturiser
10. Use as drops for ear infections

Consult your healthcare practitioner.

4. Antimony

AKA: Antimony sulphide

Ever since antimony was first discovered in ancient times to have a nourishing effect on the skin, women have been using the mineral for its beauty benefits. The mineral, which was first isolated by Italian metallurgist Vannoccio Biringuccio, is also used in cosmetics.

But antimony isn't just known for its cosmetic benefits. Centuries ago the mineral was prepared as an effective homeopathic remedy – Antimonium Crudum. This homeopathic remedy, which has a number of uses, can be used to treat skin rashes and eczema. To create the solution, the lead-grey mineral is roasted and heated with carbon to extract the antimony that lies beneath. This is then ground with lactose sugar, diluted and shaken vigorously. While the substance left behind contains virtually no traces of antimony, what is left is as an effective homeopathic treatment for skin conditions like eczema, with many studies showing antimony to have a nourishing and conditioning effect on the skin.

Consult your healthcare practitioner.

5. Apple Cider Vinegar

While it may be a popular kitchen ingredient today, the earliest recorded use of vinegar begins around 500 BC when the Babylonians used the fruit of the date palm to make wine and vinegar. European alchemists of the Middle Ages would also use vinegars flavoured with spices, herbs, fruit and flowers. In fact, any alcoholic beverage will naturally turn into vinegar. Throughout history many of these drinks would be made from fruits, vegetables and plants. The different vinegars would be used not only for pickling, drinking and flavouring, but also as medicine.

In folk remedy, apple cider vinegar is said to be an effective antiseptic, antifungal and anti-bacterial agent that relieves itching (especially itching associated with dry skin). In severe cases, a paste of cornflour and apple cider vinegar may help.

Apple cider vinegar may also be used on an itchy scalp. It is rich in malic acid, which can help kill the virus and yeast causing the problem. Acetic acid is also a natural clarifier and will lift residue from hair products and cleanse your hair at the same time. This will help keep the scalp cleaner and less likely to itch.

10 Uses for Apple Cider Vinegar

1. Lower blood pressure
2. Relief from itching
3. Aid digestion
4. Treat yeast infections
5. Help ear infections
6. Polish glass
7. Promote weight loss
8. Skin detoxification
9. Strengthen immunity
10. Restore pH balance

Apple Cider Vinegar Hair Rinse

You will need:
1/3 cup of apple cider vinegar
1 cup of water
1 or 2 drops of sage oil

Method:

1. Mix ingredients and pour into an empty spray bottle.
2. Apply evenly to your hair before shampooing.
3. Massage into your scalp for 2 to 3 minutes, rinse, shampoo and style as usual.

Consult your healthcare practitioner.

6. Apricot Kernel Oil

AKA: Prunus armeniaca

A valuable commodity on Ancient Persian trade routes, apricots have been cultivated in Persia since before the Middle Ages. Boasting a similar chemical makeup to almond oil, apricot kernel oil also features emollient-like qualities. With minerals and vitamins like A, B1, B2, B12, and C, apricot oil is great for relieving the itchy symptoms of eczema. This nourishing oil is soft on the skin and easily absorbed. While it is used less frequently than almond oil as it is more expensive to produce, apricot oil has a beautiful soothing texture and a seductive scent that is hard to resist.

Apricot Body Oil

2 parts apricot oil

1 part coconut oil

2 drops of lemon myrtle

2 drops of sage

Consult your healthcare practitioner.

7. Arsenic

AKA: *Arsenic sulphide*

While most people identify arsenic as a poison, this chemical element can also be used to treat problem skin. For more than 2,400 years arsenic, whose name was taken from the Greek word *arsenikon*, meaning 'potent', has been used as both a therapeutic agent and a poison. During the 1700s, English inventor Thomas Fowler developed a solution of arsenic trioxide in potassium bicarbonate (1 per cent weight/volume), that was used to treat asthma, chorea, eczema, pemphigus, psoriasis, anaemia, Hodgkin disease, lymphoma and leukaemia. Even Charles Darwin was a fan of the solution, using it during the 1800s in a soap form to treat eczema on his back.

However, that is not to say the use of the chemical in medicine has been without controversy. For more than 2,000 years the role of arsenic as a curative compound has been analysed and questioned. Yet despite its carcinogenicity and the toxic effects associated with long-term exposure, scientists and physicians have used it successfully in practice to treat numerous ailments and diseases.

In the Victorian times women applied arsenic powder to their faces as well as to their hair and wigs to kill lice and mites. Arsenic was also used in shampoo, reputed to help the regrowth of hair follicles. It was also thought that taking Fowlers solution, an arsenic mixture, would give them rosy fresh cheeks and so spotting opportunity British manufacturers began selling a vast array of beauty treatments. The use of arsenic powder actually caused more skin blemishes and damage, which was then covered up with more arsenic powder. Unfortunately these treatments lead to the implication of arsenic in many terrible and unnecessary deaths.

Today arsenic is no longer used in mainstream medicine to treat skin conditions; however it is still used by homeopaths to cure itches and scratches. Although arsenic is a poison, the process by which the remedy is prepared waters down the toxicity of the metal and leaves a medicinal solution. This homeopathic medicine, known as Arsenic Album, is used to treat various ailments ranging from anxiety disorders and itching to gastrointestinal complaints. In the treatment of eczema, Arsenic Album can help relieve both skin and stomach ulcers.

While working to improve the skin, Arsenic Album is said to simultaneously work to prevent leaky gut syndrome and the entry of toxins into the body. Additionally, this remedy may also reduce inflammation as well as relieve oozing lesions on the skin.

Consult your healthcare practitioner.

8. Benzoin

AKA: *Styrax benzoin*

Most common in Java, Sumatra and Thailand, benzoin is an evergreen tree that has a history in the east of being used to create incense and perfumes. An effective inhalant, benzoin found popularity as a remedy for respiratory problems. It is also useful for repairing chapped and cracked skin, as well as providing relief from itching chilblains and eczema. In western aromatherapy benzoin is regarded as a sedative, while in Chinese medicine it is believed to be a stimulant.

Benzoin is ideal for treating dry skin as it helps to improve elasticity, particularly in chapped hands and heels. Known to reduce redness, irritation and itching, benzoin also has antiseptic, astringent, carminative, deodorant, diuretic, expectorant and sedative properties.

It is recommended that you use benzoin tincture under the guidance of a health professional.

Benzoin Body Oil

You will need 20 drops of:

Flaxseed

Neroli

Benzoin

Geranium

6 vitamin E capsules

250ml coconut oil

Method:

1. Combine the ingredients in a large glass jar.
2. Add a few centimetres of water to a medium-sized saucepan and place over medium heat.
3. Screw the lid on the jar loosely and place in the saucepan.
4. As the water heats up the ingredients will begin to melt. Shake the jar to incorporate all the ingredients.
5. Pour into a decorative glass jar for storage.

Bergamot also blends well with cypress,eucalyptus, geranium, jasmine, lemon, marjoram, neroli, palmarosa, patchouli and ylang ylang.

Consult your healthcare practitioner.

9. Bergamot

AKA: Citrus bergamia

This native South East Asian tree, which was introduced to Europe by voyager Christopher Columbus, is made into an oil that can be used in everything from beverages to hand creams. Also found in the Ivory Coast, Morocco, Tunisia and Algeria, bergamot is more widely cultivated in the southern part of Italy, specifically in the coastal regions of Reggio di Calabria and Sicily. In fact, the essential oil was named after the city of Bergamo in Lombardy, Italy, where it was originally sold.

With its light and delicate texture, this refreshing oil with citrus overtones is one of the most widely used oils in perfumery. It is also one of the main ingredients in the classic 4711 Eau De Cologne and is used to flavour Earl Grey tea. The oil itself can be used to treat a range of skin conditions including acne, eczema, and psoriasis, care of its antibiotic, antiseptic, and analgesic properties.

ॐ

Bergamot Hand Cream

1 cup of distilled water

10 drops of bergamot essential oil

1 tablespoon of wax pellets

1 tablespoon of olive oil butter

¾ cup of apricot oil

2 drops of chamomile oil

2 drops of lavender oil

2 drops of sweet orange oil

Method:

1. Place the wax pellets, olive oil butter and apricot oil in a microwaveable bowl and microwave until wax pellets have melted.
2. Combine water and essential oils and add to the first bowl of ingredients.
3. Blend ingredients with a stick blender until smooth.
4. Pour into an airtight glass jar or container.

Bergamot also blends well with cypress, eucalyptus, geranium, jasmine, lemon, marjoram, neroli, palmarosa, patchouli and ylang ylang.

ॐ

Consult your healthcare practitioner.

10. Birch

AKA: Betula pubescens

Silver Birch is a tree that survives the cold climate of the northern hemisphere, growing in many countries including Scotland, England and North America. Some varieties are also now growing in temperate climate areas such as the Mediterranean. The people of northern Europe have long been very fond of this beautiful slender tree, in particular the Celts who used it as herbal medicine and for thatching and making household tools. American Indians also used birch to relieve headaches, and in poultices to treat burns and wounds and ease the pain of rheumatism.

The leaves, twigs, bark and roots are all used for medicine. In general, birch is said to have diuretic, antirheumatic, stimulant, astringent, anthelmintic, cholagogue and diaphoretic qualities.

Birch tea is often used as an ingredient in psoriasis and eczema ointments. Tea made from the tree shoots can be used as a wash for skin complaints. If the skin problem is severe, oil from the bark may be extracted through a decoction, where the bark is mashed then boiled, and used as a wash or added to a bath. Additionally, oil extracted from the buds or the bark can be used externally for acne and eczema. Both the bark and the buds can be used when antibacterial, antiviral and cell regenerative qualities are needed, making it ideal for use on many types of wounds. Today, new medicinal uses of the plant continue to be discovered.

Tincture of Birch

You will need:

2 handfuls of birch leaves

1 spoonful of chamomile flowers

1 spoonful of lavender flowers

4 cloves

Method:

1. Cover with 70 per cent alcohol.
2. Steep for three weeks, shaking now and then.
3. Strain into a dark glass bottle for storing.

It is best to take a couple of drops directly under the tongue.

The tincture can be diluted with water and the flavour disguised with honey and lemon.

Consult your healthcare practitioner.

11. Bismuth

AKA: *Bismuthinite*

B ismuth is a white, crystalline, brittle metal with a pinkish tinge. The first reference to the use of bismuth for treating skin conditions can be traced back the 18ᵗʰ century. In 1930, local treatment of eczema consisted of applying lotions and ointments with bismuth as the primary ingredient. Traditionally it was also applied in a powder form or diluted with starch or magnesia. Bismuth creams were another popular treatment at the time and were made by blending the metal with lard, cold cream or Vaseline.

Although bismuth is no longer used in mainstream medicine, the ingredient is still used in homeopathic remedies to treat eczema. According to homeopathic literature, bismuth compounds are useful in the treatment of eczema because of their absorbent, astringent and soothing properties.

Consult your healthcare practitioner.

12. Bleach Baths

Adding bleach to a bath may help control eczema's itch, however it is essential to talk with a board-certified dermatologist before beginning treatment. Never apply bleach directly to the skin and only use a weak solution and one that is not concentrated: a regular 6 per cent bleach is sufficient.

Method:

1. Use a measuring spoon to add the bleach to the bath, as directed by your dermatologist, as too much may further irritate the skin.
2. Be sure to wait until the bath is fully drawn and bleach is mixed in before you enter the tub.
3. Bathe for the recommended time – usually a maximum of 5 to 10 minutes.
4. Immediately after your bath pat your skin dry and moisturise your skin.

WARNING: Never apply bleach directly to the skin.
Consult your healthcare practitioner.

13. Borage Seed Oil

AKA: Borgao officinalis

R oman soldiers would fortify themselves with a mixture of borage tea and wine before battle. Borage also has a history of use to treat various other ailments and to improve overall health.

The borage plant is a prolific self-seeder that produces thousands of tiny little black seeds that are pressed for their oil. The borage leaves, flowers and seeds are all used as medicine. It is one of the best-known sources of gamma linolenic acid, an essential fatty acid. Borage has one of the highest amounts of the acid, making it extremely effective for dry skin and skin that is susceptible to eczema and itching. It is non-irritating oil that can still be beneficial for dry and sensitive skin.

Sipping borage tea may also help to ease stress that can contribute to itching and eczema flare-ups. The tea is easy to make. Simply chop ¼ cup borage leaves and flowers, steep in water for 10 minutes and add honey if required.

Taking borage oil twice a day in conjunction with fish oil and zinc supplements may also help treat the symptoms of eczema.

Consult your healthcare practitioner.

14. Bromelain

AKA: *Ananas comosus*

In 1493 the people of Guadeloupe first introduced Christopher Columbus to the pineapple. Later, when King Louis XIV of France bit into an unpeeled pineapple, the experience put an end to the cultivation of pineapple in France until Louis XV took over the throne in 1715. Fortunately for the natives of Central and South America, their experience has been much more positive, with people from both areas enjoying a long and rich history with the fruit.

Fresh pineapple contains bromelain, an enzyme that helps to break down protein. Bromelain was first isolated from pineapple juice in 1891 and introduced as a therapeutic supplement in 1957. The enzyme can help reduce the symptoms of both varicose veins and itchy skin. Taken with the flavonoid quercetin, it can be used to treat the itchy rashes of eczema. Additionally, pineapple contains both manganese and vitamin C, which can help reduce histamine, the chemical responsible for inflammation.

Consult your healthcare practitioner.

15. Burdock

AKA: Arctium lappa

For thousands of years the roots and leaves of the burdock plant have been used to treat rheumatism, gout, and skin disorders such as psoriasis. Used in Native American medicine, burdock was also a valued herb during the Middle Ages.

Burdock has an ancient and respected reputation as a nutritive liver tonic that helps to clean and build the blood, while its diuretic properties (ability to increase the frequency of urination) helps in the elimination of waste materials.

Taken internally, this root promotes sweating and the elimination of harmful high levels of uric acid via the kidneys. Burdock tea is suitable for any skin condition that benefits from detoxification. It also blends well with dandelion root as a tonic drink for the liver.

Burdock has antifungal, anti-bacterial and anti-tumour properties. As such, it can be used to treat chronic skin disorders like eczema and psoriasis.

Burdock Salve

You will need:

Grated burdock root

Almond oil

Beeswax

Method:

1. Place grated burdock into the almond oil in a pyrex dish and cover.
2. Put the dish in a pan with hot water and heat to 200°C for 2-3 hours.
3. Strain the liquid and return to pyrex dish with beeswax. Add more beeswax to make a thicker salve.
4. Pour into small, clean jars.

Consult your healthcare practitioner.

16. Calendula

AKA: *Calendula officinalis*

Calendua is mentioned in the ancient medical books. Albertus Magnus in the 17th century wrote that calendula was an excellent healer. The Greeks and Romans used the golden calendula in many rituals and ceremonies. The name calendula has been derived from the word 'calendar' as the plant bears flowers in all the months of the year.

This herb has been known for many generations as an anti-inflammatory agent that can treat a range of different skin conditions. Calendula is believed to benefit eczema by reducing inflammation, eliminating bacteria and helping the skin heal. One study in 2004 found that the occurrence of acute dermatitis in women who had undergone radiation treatment for breast cancer was significantly lower for those who had used calendula ointment.

The calendula oil is obtained by infusing calendula's orange petals in carrier oil in order to extract its properties. This process is known as maceration. Calendula is famous for its great skin healing properties and can be used to treat bruises, cuts and skin irritations. It is also ideal for itchy, chapped and dry skin.

Calendula Ointment

You will need:

½ cup of calendula petals

½ cup of chamomile flowers

4 drops of lavender oil

¾ cup of olive oil

¼ cup of grated beeswax or beeswax pastilles

Cheesecloth for straining

Heavy base saucepan

Mixing spoon

Measuring cup

Rubber band

Method:

1. Place calendula leaves, chamomile flowers and olive oil into saucepan and warm slowly for 3 hours.
2. A rubber band will secure the cheesecloth while you strain the mixture into a bowl.
3. Stir in lavender drops and beeswax until melted.

Pour into a clean jar and seal well.

Consult your healthcare practitioner.

17. Camphor

AKA: Cinnamomum camphora

Camphor has been used medicinally since 600 AD. Camphor oil is derived from the camphor laurel tree native to China and Japan. This white crystalline substance with a strong odour and pungent taste has been used for centuries in oil form to treat skin conditions such as itching and irritations.

Made by distilling the bark and wood of the camphor tree, the oil can serve as an air freshener, moth repellent, embalming fluid and as a medicine. Camphor has been used in Chinese medicine for centuries to treat arthritis and other muscle aches and pains. It may also be used as a vapour for coughs and colds.

Although an effective treatment, camphor oil should never be used on broken skin. In the 1950s camphor was given as an oral treatment for itching and eczema and was shown to cause bowel and intestinal problems.

Camphor appears to stimulate nerve endings that relieve symptoms such as pain and itching when applied to the skin. However, in some cases it may cause the skin to dry out and as such it may not be suitable to treat eczema. The application of camphor oil is arguably more suited to an itch from insect bites like mosquito.

ॐ

Camphor Mosquito Spray

You will need:

Eucalyptus oil

Clove oil

Camphor oil

Method:

1. Fill a spray bottle with water.
2. Add 4 drops of each oil.
3. Shake well before using.

Another way to repel mosquitoes is to place camphor tablets in a warm place inside a room. The tablets will evaporate into the air and keep the room mosquito free.

ॐ

Consult your healthcare practitioner.

18. Carrot Oil

AKA: *Daucus carota*

The earliest vegetable definitely known to be a carrot dates back to the 10th century. Carrot seed oil is extracted from Daucuscarota of the Apiaceae family and is also known as 'wild carrot'. Cultivated carrots also belong to the Daucus carota family. The name carrot is derived from the Greek word 'Caroton' and it had great medicinal value in ancient times. Carrot was mentioned by Greek and Latin writers by various names but it was Galen who called it Daucus to distinguish it from the parsnip.

Carrot seed oil contains a wide range of antioxidants including a carotenoid called Beta-carotene. It also has many other carotenoids and antioxidant including vitamin A and vitamin E. Vitamin A nourishes the skin and one of the most concentrated sources of the nutrient is carrot oil.

When externally applied carrot seed can help sooth itchy skin and is thought to be helpful in treating eczema. It can help relieve skin infections and open wounds. It also tones the skin and slows down the signs of aging. It is used in many cosmetics and skincare products.

Carrot Body Oil

You will need:

20 drops of carrot oil

12 drops of neroli oil

6 drops of frankincense

4 drops of lavender

8 vitamin E capsules

250ml olive oil

Blend the oils together and store in an air-tight container.

Carrot Seed Oil Scrub

You will need:

1 cup of sea salt

5 drops of carrot seed oil

5 drops of calendula oil

5 drops of lavender oil

Almond oil to cover

Method

1. Blend together gently and store in a container by your bath.
2. Use a scoopful when bathing.

Carrot oil blends well with bergamot, juniper, lavender, lemon, lime and cedarwood.

Consult your healthcare practitioner.

19. Cedarwood

AKA: *Juniperus virginiana, Cedrus atlantica*

The use of the cedar tree for medicinal purposes goes as far back as biblical times. The Egyptians used the oil in cosmetics, incense and as an insect repellent, while Native Americans used cedarwood in medicine and purification rituals.

The antiseptic, anti-seborrheic and mild astringent properties of cedarwood make it a popular choice for treating dandruff and for relieving scalp itchiness. Cedarwood oil can minimise the peeling of the skin and by regularizing sebum production, reduce any itching that occurs.

It can be used to treat eczema, psoriasis, acne, scabies, and wounds.

Consult your healthcare practitioner.

20. Chamomile Oil

AKA: Anthemis nobilis or Matricaria recutita

There are two different chamomiles, Roman and German, and both contain antibacterial, antifungal, anti-inflammatory and antiseptic properties. Good chamomile oil is macerated containing either German or Roman chamomile flowers. Chamomile is considered to be hypoallergenic, with the ability to neutralise skin irritants. It is one of the few herbs that have been included in clinical trials as a means of examining its effectiveness in skincare.

Clinical trials have also shown chamomile to reduce the incidence of dermatitis: in one trial chamomile ointment was found to be effective in reducing dermatitis following a single application of sodium lauryl sulfate.

Chamomile Anti-itch Salve

Blend cocoa butter, shea nut butter, coconut oil, jojoba oil with a few drops of chamomile, myrrh, frankincense and rose.

Consult your healthcare practitioner.

21. Chickweed

AKA: Stellaria media

Not a commonly known herb, chickweed is a small white flower that is native to Europe. It has been used in herbal medicine and Chinese medicine for hundreds of years – even today it is still recommended by herbalists for skin diseases. It has been known to soothe severe itching where all other remedies have failed. This little herb exhibits extremely effective anti-inflammatory and anti-viral activity, which is due to the number of compounds it contains, including polysaccharides, flavonoids and cyclic peptides.

The whole plant can be used internally or externally. Chickweed can be added to salads or you can steam the leaves or boil the stems as a vegetable. Taken as a tincture or tea, it has a reputation as a remedy for rheumatism.

An infusion of the fresh or dried plant can be added to bath water and its emollient qualities will help to reduce inflammation.

Chickweed oil combines well with other herbal infused oils like yarrow oil or St John's Wort oil. It is an ingredient in many commercial skin care products.

Chickweed Salve

You will need:

A small jar

1 cup of chickweed

1 cup of olive oil

1/8 cup of beeswax

½ teaspoon vitamin E oil

Method:

1. Place the chickweed into the jar and cover with the olive oil.
2. Make sure you get all the air bubbles out.
3. Place the lid on and let it sit for 2 weeks. Shake once a day.
4. After 2 weeks strain the oil into a saucepan.
5. Add in the beeswax and vitamin E oil and gently heat until beeswax has melted.
6. Pour into small containers and let the salve set.

You can add a few drops of essential oils like lavender, chamomile, comfrey, sweet orange and rosemary to the salve mixture.

Consult your healthcare practitioner.

22. Cleavers

AKA: Galium aparine

This herb has a long history of use in skincare. Otherwise known as goosegrass, cleavers has astringent properties and is thought to have a toning, firming effect on skin. When used externally, cleavers is said to benefit eczema and psoriasis thanks to its anti-inflammatory properties. It is extremely gentle and is believed to have an influence on the lymphatic system, which may help the body react better to the presence of eczema. Cleavers is also used externally for healing wounds and sores, cysts, boils, swellings and for treating skin infections and swollen lymph glands.

You can create a gentle herbal tea skin wash using organic cleavers. To treat your itch, gently pat the skin or bathe it with the tea blend.

Consult your healthcare practitioner.

23. Coal Tar

Tars and resins have been used as a treatment for skin problems for more than 2,000 years. Coal tar is obtained by the destructive distillation of bituminous coal at very high temperatures. It is most often obtained in solution form and mixed with other ingredients, such as salicylic acid and sulphur to make lotions, creams, ointments and shampoos. Some patients who use these products have found the tar odour to be offensive and complain about it staining their clothes.

Coal tar is thought to correct the defect of differentiation in keratinocytes (the predominant cell type in the epidermis or the outermost layer of the skin), of patients with psoriasis. The use of coal tar products has dropped significantly since the introduction of new herbal formulas in creams that are more practical and less offensive on the nose.

Consult your healthcare practitioner.

24. Coconut Oil

Coconut oil or copra oil is an edible oil extracted from the kernel or meat of matured coconuts harvested from the coconut palm. It has various uses in both food and medicine industries. In a study coconut oil and mineral oil showed comparable effects. Both oils were effective in improving the skin's hydration levels and increasing the levels of lipids, a group of naturally occurring molecules on the skin's surface. With no significant difference in TEWL (transepidermal water loss) and skin pH (acid levels), the treatment was deemed safe. Subjective grading by the investigators and visual analogue scales used by the patients showed a general trend toward better improvement with coconut oil than with mineral oil.

Patients with atopic dermatitis have inflamed skin with defects in the epidermal (outermost layer of the skin) and barrier function, primarily related to inflammation and dehydration, which leads them to use ostensibly soothing moisturisers. Most mass market skin care products however contain mineral oil and related petrochemical ingredients, which not only may contribute to skin irritation, but more serious skin conditions such as skin cancer, as well as bodily accumulation of significant quantities in organs. This is why natural, food-quality ingredients like coconut oil, which have been used in traditional cultures for thousands of years, hold great promise as a viable alternative and are increasingly becoming the subject of modern scientific investigation.

Organic Coconut Oil Body Lotion

You will need:

A small saucepan

½ cup of organic almond oil

¼ cup of organic coconut oil

¼ cup of organic beeswax

4 drops of chamomile oil

4 drops of lavender oil

Method:

1. Slowly heat the oil mixture.
2. Stir in beeswax until melted.
3. Pour into a small jar and use within 6 months.

Consult your healthcare practitioner.

25. Comfrey

AKA: Symphytum officinale

Also known as 'knit-bone', comfrey is a great skin healing herb. Comfrey is said to help knit cells back together after a laceration or abrasion. It contains a cosmeceutical called allantoin that is used to treat wounds, ulcers, burns, sunburn, eczema, psoriasis, impetigo and acne, as well as other skin eruptions.

The chemical compound found in comfrey, known as allantoin, works as an antioxidant and encourages the regeneration of new cells in addition to speeding up the shedding process of dead cells. With its skin softening properties, comfrey is also said to act as a remover of scaly tissue.

Consult your healthcare practitioner.

26. Cumin Seed Oil

AKA: Cuminum cyminum

Perhaps most familiar in curries, cumin seeds are cold pressed for their oil. Although frequently used in cooking, it is also known for its cosmetic properties and is thought to be effective in the treatment of eczema and other skin irritations.

Treating eczema with black cumin oil leads to surprisingly quick results. Black cumin oil soothes the itch, stabilizes the immune system and supports the healing of the infected skin areas. Cumin seed oil may also be used as an effective treatment for neurodermatitis.

Cumin Eczema Treatment

Mix 1 teaspoon of cumin oil, 1 tablespoon of manuka honey and 1 tablespoon of extra virgin olive oil.

Apply the paste twice day.

Consult your healthcare practitioner.

27. Cypress

AKA: *Cupressus sempervirens*

C ypress comes from the Greek word 'semper vivens' meaning 'live forever.' Some indigenous people were known to have burnt cypress wood to ward off mosquitoes and midges. The tree is a perennial and originated from the East. Now it is mostly found in gardens and cemeteries in the Mediterranean region.

Ancient cultures practiced the art of making essential oils by first soaking the flowers, bark, twigs and leaves in oil for a period of time. They would then use linens to filter, purify and isolate the oils for a concentrated and potent form.

The oil has a refreshing pine-needle aroma and is often used in antiseptic creams and lotions. With astringent, antiseptic, antispasmodic, deodorant and diuretic properties, it can be used to treat itching: in certain cases it is more effective than some medications. Use it on affected areas to soothe irritation.

❧

Cypress Body Wash

You will need:

A mixing bowl and spoon

6 tablespoons of liquid castile soap

4 tablespoons of honey

3 tablespoons of olive oil

3 tablespoons of coconut oil

10 drops of cypress oil

Method:

1. Combine the mixture gently.
2. Pour into a plastic bottle to use in the shower.

Castile soap is traditionally made from olive oil and is named after the Castile region in Spain where the people used to make the soap from their olives. There are no petro-chemicals or sulphates in Castile soap. Liquid Castile soap retains its glycerine which is a natural humectant or moisturiser due to its water binding capabilities.

❧

Consult your healthcare practitioner.

28. Diet

Food allergies are a common cause of allergic skin reactions and occur when the body incorrectly identifies certain foods as a hazard. When the body or the immune system recognises something to be harmful, it will develop antibodies to fight it off.

Today, more and more people are experiencing food allergies. While there are many theories as to why this is occurring, no cause has been successfully identified. One of these theories is that the preservative used in vaccinations may be responsible: for example, it has been suggested that the albumin or proteins in vaccines may cause egg allergies. Recently, two studies have linked meat and wheat consumption during pregnancy with eczema in babies.

Whatever the cause, our gut has a lot to do with food allergies. One or more food items irritating our gastrointestinal tract can trigger an allergic reaction because of inflammation.

Even though food allergies can occur at any age, certain allergens are more common in different age brackets. Clinical studies have shown that hens' eggs and cows' milk are the most common allergens in young sensitive infants. In older children, adolescents and adults, inhaled allergens and pollen-related foods more commonly cause allergic reactions.

Certain food items can cause eczema to flare up. Although it appears on the skin, eczema needs to be treated from within, in addition to attending to external symptoms. Eczema can be treated internally by making dietary changes and/or taking herbs and supplements, and externally by applying soothing lotions and healing potions. A candida albicans (yeast) overgrowth in the gastrointestinal tract can be a trigger for eczema. This can be improved with a change in diet.

Despite the many dietary triggers that can cause allergic reactions, there are eight foods that have been identified as the main culprits. These include: eggs, fish, milk, tree nuts, peanuts, wheat, soy and shellfish, which account for 90 per cent of all reactions. According to the food allergy network, peanuts are the leading cause of severe food allergy reactions, with as many as one-third of peanut-sensitive patients experiencing severe reactions, such as near-fatal and fatal anaphylaxis.

Other food items – including gluten, dairy products, corn, beans, lentils, meats such as pork chicken and beef, as well as coffee, citrus fruit and nightshade vegetables – can cause reactions ranging from mild itching and irritations of the skin to severe anaphylaxis. Be sure to carefully read food labels.

Consult your healthcare practitioner.

29. Echinacea

AKA: *Echinacea angustifolia*

The name of this fascinating plant is derived from the Greek word 'echinos,' meaning hedgehog. This plant has a long tradition of use amongst North American Indian tribes where the herb was used as an antibiotic, antiseptic, decongestant and tonic. European settlers brought Echinacea back to Europe, where it quickly became a popular herbal remedy.

The main virtue of echinacea is its anti-microbial power against bacteria, fungi and viruses. Chemical analysis of echinacea reveals a fascinating combination of substances, including some with anti-viral and anti-cancer properties and others that regenerate tissue.

This herb is useful in ointments and extracts for the treatment of wounds, minor burns, cuts and mouth sores. A tincture of echinacea can be applied to skin conditions on a bandage to help relieve itching and inflammation caused by eczema or psoriasis.

☙

Echinacea Soothing Balm

You will need:

3 tablespoons of almond oil

3 tablespoons of shea nut butter

6 drops of echinacea oil

6 drops of chamomile oil

Beeswax to thicken

Method:

1. Combine the ingredients in a glass bowl.

2. Place the bowl over a saucepan of hot water.

3. Stir in beeswax to thicken.

4. Once combined pour into a glass jar.

A combination of soothing essential oils like lavender, benzoin and cedarwood can also be used in the soothing balm.

☙

Consult your healthcare practitioner.

30. Elderberry

AKA: Sambucus nigra

Elderberry, also known as elderflower, is a tree that bears cream-coloured flowers and dark purple berries in autumn. The name *elder* is likely to be derived from the Anglo-Saxon word 'aeld', meaning fire. Elderberry trees are native to Europe but have been naturalised in the Americas and other countries. They have a long history of medicinal use, particularly in England, where the berries are commonly used to make elderberry wine and pies. (Once upon a time the elderberry was even referred to as 'nature's medicine chest.') The use of the berries as a purgative dates back to Hippocrates.

In Victorian times, distilled elderflower water was used as highly valued emollient. It was also said that if a man and woman drank together from elderflower-infused ale, they would marry within a year.

Traditionally elderberry has been used to relieve pain, inflammation, water retention and congestion. All parts of the elderberry tree, including the bark, flowers and leaves, have been used in herbal medicine. The leaves can be added to topical creams and baths to treat inflammatory disorders such as arthritis, boils and eczema. Long used for bruises, chilblains and various skin irritations, an infusion of elderflowers can be added to bath water for a refreshing wash that soothes irritable nerves and relieves itchy skin.

Elderflower water may also be sprayed onto skin to relieve itching.

∽
℘

Elderflower Water

You will need:

2 cups of elderflowers

A stainless steel saucepan

½ teaspoon of vodka for preserving

Distilled water

Spray bottle

Method:

1. Place the elderflowers in the saucepan and cover with distilled water.

2. Cover and heat to simmer.

3. Turn the heat down as low as it will go.

4. Continue to heat for around 10 minutes.

5. Turn off the heat and allow the mixture to sit overnight to infuse.

6. Strain twice through a muslin cloth.

7. Add the vodka to preserve and bottle for storage.

∽
℘

Consult your healthcare practitioner.

31. Environment

The naturally therapeutic effect of climate and weather was recognised as far back as the Sumerian-Babylonian era around 2000 BC. Pre-Socratic philosophers reference the positive effect of sunbathing in their writing. Hippocrates (460-377 BC) wrote about it in his epidemic books, which concern the influence of seasons and atmospheric conditions.

In patients with atopic eczema, certain ranges of thermos-hydric (temperature and water) atmosphere conditions are ideal. A balance of heat and water loss on the skin's surface is also essential for the skin to feel comfortable.

For many people, extremely cold environments can cause eczema to flare when the skin becomes too dry. Moisturisers are an important eczema treatment, especially in cold weather. They help prevent skin from drying out, cracking and itching. In the winter, a moisturising ointment is most effective in preventing moisture loss. The use of a humidifier to add moisture to dry indoor air is also recommended.

Several environmental factors can cause itches and scratches. Some possible environmental triggers for adult eczema include: dry heat, cold weather, emotional stress, wool clothing, dust mites, detergents, perfumed lotions, sweating and pollens.

Dust mites are near-microscopic mites that live in fabrics and mattresses, attached to dust. People who have eczema are likely to have an allergy to dust mites. Several steps may be taken to minimise eczema that is caused by dust mites:

- Use mite proof covers for your mattresses (be sure to wash these every 1-2 weeks)
- Use hardwood flooring and avoid cloth furniture in the bedroom
- Use synthetic pillows
- When you dust the room, 'wet dust' it
- Vacuum the bedroom floor and mattresses every week
- Air the house out regularly
- Restrict the amount of soft toys
- Maintain a low humidity where possible to keep dust mites to a minimum.

Pets can be another source of misery for some people with eczema. The dander or dead skin that the animals shed is a common allergen and is linked to eczema and itching. If there is no evidence a pet is causing an exacerbation of symptoms, there's no need to permanently get rid of the pet – at least not yet.

One option is to have a friend, relative or even a pet kennel 'babysit' your beloved pet for a few days. While it is away, you can observe whether there is any improvement in your condition. If you do see an improvement, the pet is almost certainly a factor and unfortunately, it may be better if you said goodbye to your furry friend.

Pollen is another environmental factor that can cause some eczema sufferers grief. In fact, this is one of the most common sources of misery from itching and sneezing. At times the immune system misinterprets and attacks pollen as a dangerous invader, causing all kinds of discomfort, including itching and eczema.

Having a pollen allergy on a beautiful day is no fun; you know that if you venture out, you will have to pay for it. If you do choose to go outside, make sure you cover up and wash the pollen off your skin when you return, to minimise your reaction.

Mould, a fungus that grows both inside the home and in the open, can also cause eczema. Mould spores, which are very light and fly through the air, can cause a reaction on the skin when deposited on someone who is sensitive to it. Unfortunately all that is needed for mould to thrive is high humidity, so to keep mould in check, make sure there are no water leaks in your home. Lowering humidity can also help.

Lastly, if you are sensitive to chlorine in water, swimming can also cause itchy episodes. To swim without a reaction, bathe or wash the chlorine off the skin immediately after exiting the pool. Then apply a moisturiser, as dry skin tends to intensify the itchy feeling. Before taking a dip, dabbing a petroleum-based jelly like Vaseline on the worst areas can also help.

32. Eucalyptus

AKA: Eucalyptus globulus

Although it is indigenous to Australia, the eucalyptus tree is now grown worldwide. The tree's oil has a long history among the aboriginal population of Australia and has been used for centuries. Thanks to its many proven properties, it is now grown in countries like the United States of America, China and Russia. Eucalyptus oil is derived from the leaves of the Australian fever tree or blue gum tree. The oil is antimicrobial, antifungal, antibacterial, antiviral and anti-inflammatory.

It is useful for skin problems and may prevent the bacterial growth that can slow down wounds and tissue from healing. The oil also seems to improve inflamed cuts, wounds and ulcers. A mixture of olive oil and eucalyptus oil may help relieve itching. You can also add a drop or two of the oil into your bathwater to ease the effects of skin infections.

Eucalyptus Itch Relief Spray

You will need:

I cup of olive oil

1 cup of aloe vera juice

1 teaspoon of eucalyptus oil

1 teaspoon of grapeseed oil

1 teaspoon of jojoba oil

8 vitamin E capsules

Method:

Combine the mixture and pour into a spray bottle.
This also works as a preventative.

Consult your healthcare practitioner.

33. Evening Primrose Oil

AKA: Oenothera biennis

Although Native Americans used the seeds for food and the whole plant to heal bruises, evening primrose oil (EPO) has only recently been used as medicine. European settlers took the root back to England and Germany, where it was eaten as food. Much like borage oil, evening primrose oil is rich in unsaturated fatty acids that repair and maintain skin tissue. This oil is frequently used in cosmetic preparations and is suitable for dry skin.

Evening primrose oil is used mostly to relieve the itchiness caused by certain skin conditions, such as eczema and dermatitis. It is very high in essential fatty acids, in particular gamma linolenic acid or GLA.

GLA may reduce inflammation in the skin and therefore reduce swelling and redness in the skin. The antioxidant effect of GLA also relieves itching and prevents flaking.

The usual recommended doses of evening primrose oil vary between 2 grams and 8 grams per day. This will help plump up cellular membranes, repair old cells and construct new cells in the skin.

Alternatively, a tincture or an infusion made with one teaspoon of the plant to one cup of water may be used. Evening primrose oil is not recommended for epileptics or pregnant and breastfeeding women.

ॐ

Evening Primrose Oil Calming Ointment

This is an ointment that has to be made and used each week. Evening primrose can oxidise quickly. Please store in a cool place like your refrigerator.

You will need:
1 tablespoon evening primrose oil
1 tablespoon borage oil
1 tablespoon vitamin E oil
1 tablespoon coconut oil
1 tablespoon calendula oil
1 tablespoon chamomile oil

Method:

Combine all the oils together in a spray bottle.
Shake well before applying. Store in a cool place.

ॐ

Consult your healthcare practitioner.

34. Fish Oil

AKA: EPA

A rich source of omega-3 fatty acids, fish oil can be used to treat a number of medical conditions. In one study, people taking fish oil equal to 1.8 grams of EPA (one of the omega-3 fatty acids found in fish oil) experienced significant reduction in symptoms of eczema after 12 weeks. The theory is that fish oil helps to reduce leukotriene B4, an inflammatory substance that plays a role in eczema.

Talk to your doctor before taking fish oil, especially if you are taking any blood-thinning medications or are looking to take a high dose. If you're taking high dose fish oil, make sure you use a brand that removes most of the vitamin A, as too much over time can become toxic.

Consult your healthcare practitioner.

35. Flavonoids

Flavonoids are a group of plant metabolites (substances produced during metabolism) believed to be beneficial for their cell signalling pathways and antioxidant effects. These molecules are found in a variety of fruits and vegetables and are the major colouring agent in plants (particularly dark berries).

In skin and other parts of the body, flavonoid action works against cancer and is anti-inflammatory, keeping the skin's stress loads down and strengthening connective tissue. One flavonoid called quercetin can help alleviate eczema, sinusitis, asthma and hay fever.

Some good sources of flavonoids are red wine, dark chocolate and tea, as well as coloured fruit and vegetables (particularly parsley, onions, blueberries, and bananas).

Consult your healthcare practitioner.

36. Frankincense

AKA: Boswellia carterii

Frankincense originates from the Middle East and together with myrrh, was the first gum to be used in incense. This aromatic resin gets its name from the word 'franc', which means luxuriant or 'real incense'.

In Ancient Egypt, Egyptians used frankincense as an offering to the Gods and as an ingredient in their rejuvenating facemasks. It was also used to fumigate the sick, banish evil spirits, and purify the soul. But perhaps it was the Hebrews who valued frankincense most of all, offering it as a gift to the baby Jesus.

This haunting fragrance is spicy and produces feelings of calm and serenity. The aroma is soothing for the mind and can be used to calm anxious and obsessive people. Frankincense is an excellent skin tonic and can be used for healing and to prevent scarring. It also eases inflammation and itching. The resin may be used in a base cream for easy application.

Frankincense and Rose Anti-Itch Cream

You will need:

3 tablespoons of almond oil

3 tablespoons of shea nut butter

Beeswax to thicken

2 drops of rose oil

2 drops of frankincense oil

Method:

1. Combine the ingredients in a glass bowl.

2. Place the bowl over a saucepan of hot water.

3. Stir in the beeswax to thicken.

4. Once combined, pour into a glass jar.

Feel free to replace the almond oil with safflower or coconut oil to cut down on the amount of nut oils in the cream.

Consult your healthcare practitioner.

37. Fumitory

AKA: *Fumaria officinalis*

The fumitory plant takes its name from the appearance of its flowers, which closely resemble smoke rising from the ground. Preferring sunny environments, fumitory best grows in light, well-drained soil. Found in France, Spain, Austria, Asia and the UK, almost all of this plant, including the stems, roots and flowers, can be used as healing remedies.

Used since Roman times, this plant had a prominent place in the herbal medicine of medieval and 18th century Europe – more so than it does today. It has a history of being taken internally and applied externally to cure itching, purify the blood and aid the spleen and liver. It has also been used to 'heal the skin, clear madness and the frenzies, and to scare the tan from summer's cheek'.

Because of fumitory's anti-inflammatory qualities, it works well for treating both eczema and psoriasis. Its effectiveness may be due to its diuretic and purgative actions, which have a general cleansing effect on the whole body. It contains antioxidants and fatty acids that heal the skin, and up to 30 alkaloids, substances that often have strong pharmaceutical actions.

Fumitory Compress

Infusions of essential oils are very effective as compresses. Chemical analysis of the fumitory has shown that when compressed, its leaves give out a juice that contains therapeutic qualities. A compress can be made with a cloth or bandage. Fold the cloth or bandage into a pad and soak it in the herbal infusion.

You will need:

Dried fumitory leaves

Cloth or bandage

A bowl

Boiling water

Method:

1. Place 2 teaspoons of dried fumitory leaves in a cup of boiling water and allow it to infuse for 10 to 15 minutes.
2. Soak the cloth pad or bandage in the infusion.
3. Apply 2 to 3 times a day.

Fumitory Infusion

Put 2 teaspoons of dried flowers into 150ml of boiling water. Infuse for 10 minutes and strain.

Consult your healthcare practitioner.

38. Geranium

AKA: Pelargonium graveolens

Ever since the Ancient Greeks and Egyptians first used it to promote beautiful and radiant skin, geranium oil has been a popular ingredient in alternative medicine. Also used by North American Indian tribes, geranium in the Victorian era was often kept in parlours where fresh leaves were always available to revive the senses.

For centuries it was also planted around cottages to ward off evil spirits. Geraniums are fragrant all year long and their scent is released when you crush the small beads of oil contained at the base of the leaf hairs. The most popular scented geranium during the Victorian times was the rose scented geranium.

Gentle on the skin, geranium oil can be used by almost everybody, anywhere, anytime. For centuries the plant was also planted around cottages to ward off evil spirits.

Helping to balance sebum, a fatty secretion that keeps skin supple, geranium is handy for treating both eczema and fungal problems. Apply a couple of drops to a cotton ball to treat the problem area.

Geranium and Rose Hand Cream

You will need:

2 tablespoons of almond oil

2 tablespoons of jojoba oil

2 tablespoons of coconut oil

Beeswax to thicken

6 drops of calendula oil

4 drops of chamomile oil

4 drops of geranium oil

2 drops of rose oil

Method:

1. Combine the ingredients in a glass bowl.

2. Place the bowl over a saucepan of hot water.

3. Stir in the beeswax to thicken.

4. Once combined, pour into a glass jar.

Consult your healthcare practitioner.

39. Goat Milk

Thought to be one of the first domesticated animals, goats have a long history of providing humans with nourishment through their milk and meat, with the earliest remnants of domesticated goats dating back 10,000 years.

Today goat milk baths are a popular beauty treatment, however Cleopatra is thought to have started the trend back in Ancient Egypt, although it is unclear whether she used goat or donkey milk – or a mixture of both. The Roman Emperor Nero's wife, Poppaea Sabina, is also said to have loved a dip in the white liquid.

Nourishing for the skin, goat milk baths heal rough and damaged patches while encouraging new skin cells to grow. The unique protein structure of goat milk, with its much shorter protein strands, is easily absorbed into the skin. It also contains many natural minerals and vitamins.

There are many benefits from using goat soap. Goat soap can help to slow down the signs of aging due to its high content of alpha-hydroxy acids. It can also reduce inflammation thanks to its fat molecule content, in addition to soothing dry and damaged skin. Packed full of essential nutrients and vitamins D, C, B1, B6, B12 and E, goat soap is high in selenium, a mineral known for its antioxidant qualities.

ॐ

Goat Milk and Honey Bath

You will need:

2 tablespoons of baking soda

1 cup of boiling water

1 cup of honey

4 cups of goat milk

1 teaspoon of chamomile oil

A mixing bowl

Method:

1. Incorporate all the ingredients in a bowl.
2. Mix well and pour into your bath.

Chamomile oil could replace calendula oil.

ॐ

Consult your healthcare practitioner.

40. Goldenseal

AKA: *Hydrastis canadensis*

Long used by Native Americans, the Cherokee tribe and others would mix this herb with bear fat to repel insects. First introduced to Europe during 1760, goldenseal later went on to become a favourite among Victorian herbalists.

Goldenseal contains the chemical berberine, which may be effective against bacteria and fungi. This herb has been used to treat wounds, herpes sores, and other skin conditions. With its anti-inflammatory, antimicrobial, antiseptic and astringent properties, it can be used to ease the inflammation and itching caused by skin irritations like eczema. Infusions of goldenseal powder are also used as a treatment for psoriasis. Goldenseal is currently being researched for its possible immune stimulation qualities.

Taking goldenseal over a long period of time can reduce absorption of B vitamins. It should be avoided during pregnancy and lactation, and if you suffer from gastrointestinal inflammation.

Some herbalists urge caution when you are choosing your goldenseal products because they may be unsustainably sourced as opposed to being organically grown.

☙

Goldenseal Salve

You will need:

1 cup of organic olive oil

1/4 cup of grated beeswax

4 vitamin E capsules

6 drops of goldenseal essential oil

Method:

1. Combine the ingredients in a glass bowl.
2. Place the bowl over a saucepan of hot water.
3. Puncture the vitamin E capsules and add to mixture.
4. Stir in the beeswax to thicken.
5. Once combined, pour into a small glass jar.

☙

Consult your healthcare practitioner.

41. Gotu Kola

AKA: *Centella asiatica*

F ew medicinal plants have as long a history of use as gotu kola. In Chinese medicine it is listed among the 'miracle elixirs of life.' A centrepiece of the traditional Hindu medicine, Ayurveda, it has been used for thousands of years to treat infected wounds, eczema, psoriasis and lupus rash.

While it is most famous for its blood vessel strengthening properties, gotu kola is also a diuretic and can be used to manage a variety of health problems. Ayurveda practitioners recommend the use of gotu kola to treat eczema, psoriasis, epilepsy, intermittent fevers, hair loss and bowel disorders. It is also believed to improve memory, increase longevity and boost the immune system, in addition to being an effective adrenal and blood purifier.

In terms of skincare, gotu kola has shown great promise in the treatment of eczema and psoriasis. Known to stimulate collagen synthesis, this plant may be good news for those seeking rejuvenated skin – and science backs this up. When creams containing oil and water extracts of the leaves were administered each morning to seven eczema patients, five patients displayed complete clearance of lesions within three to seven weeks. One patient experienced clearance of almost all of their lesions. Although this study was not controlled, a placebo effect was considered unlikely. Experience indicated that the cream was non-toxic and cosmetically acceptable, making it suitable for long-term use.

$\approx$

10 Benefits of Using Gotu Kola:

1. Wound healing
2. Eczema relief
3. Lessen stretch marks
4. Dermatitis relief
5. Reduce thread veins
6. Relieve varicose veins
7. Maintain healthy skin
8. Strengthen arteries
9. Reduce scarring
10. Improve circulation

$\approx$

Consult your healthcare practitioner.

42. Heartsease

AKA: *Viola tricolour*

Although part of the violet family, heartsease is more than just a pretty flower. One of the several variants of violet, heartsease is an annual or short-lived perennial plant found in Europe. Growing up to fifteen centimetres, this beautiful wild flower blooms from April to September and comes in shades of blue, yellow, purple and white. It is abundant in Vitamin C, beta-carotene, salicylic acid, cyclotides, Saponins, phenolic glycosides and flavonoids.

Considered as a blood purifier, heartsease is associated with the treatment of a variety of skin problems including acne, eczema, dermatitis, psoriasis and other itches. Viola tricolour can be used internally both as a compress or ointment in the treatment of eczema, psoriasis and acne. It is also a suitable remedy for clearing cradle cap in babies.

Herbal tea made from two parts agrimony and chamomile and one part stinging nettle and heartsease can be taken three times a day to soothe itching. In addition to drinking the tea, it may also be applied as a compress to and applied to problem areas.

Consult your healthcare practitioner.

43. Hemp Seed Oil

AKA: Cannabis sativa

Throughout history hemp seed oil has long been used as a medicine – but don't worry, it doesn't contain any psychoactive properties. Egyptologists agree that the *Eber's Papyrus* (the earliest complete medical textbook known to exist) makes several references to hemp seed oil and its use in treating inflammation.

In fact, hemp seed oil is another rich source of essential fatty acids and has been found to provide relief from the itchy symptoms of eczema. Full of nutrients, hemp seed oil contains only a small trace amount of THC (delta-9-tetrahydrocannabinol), the cannabinoid responsible for inducing the 'high' when consuming cannabis.

A clinical study in Finland documented a remarkable reduction in dryness and itching, and an overall improvement in symptoms, when it was used on eczema sufferers.

Consult your healthcare practitioner.

44. Homeopathy

How does homeopathy work? The answer to this question is not fully known. Founded by German physician Samuel Hahnemann in 1796, homeopathy is an alternative medicine that is still used today. Hahnemann believed medicine that caused a mild nausea in a healthy person would cure a sick one.

The powerful effect of the very diluted remedies used in homeopathy is a puzzling subject for researchers. Many dilutions are so high that no molecular trace of the original substance can be found. It is thought that the properties of a correct homeopathic remedy for an ailment in some way resonate with and strengthen the body's efforts to realign its unbalanced energy flows.

Homeopathic combinations, when used as directed and with proven remedies, are safe and can be effective, with rarely any side effects. You can feel confident that this approach, which has been used for over two hundred years, can effectively stimulate the immune system rather than diminish it. Before prescribing a remedy, homeopaths take into account a person's constitutional type, which includes their physical self, emotional self and psychological makeup. An experienced homeopath assesses all of these factors when determining the most effective treatment for each individual. Homeopathy, whether used in combination or as a single remedy, can assist the body in rediscovering its natural ability to heal itself.

⚘

Homeopathy can be used to treat a wide range of illnesses such as:

1. Allergies
2. Atopic dermatitis
3. Arthritis
4. Irritable bowel syndrome
5. Muscle sprains
6. Headaches and migraine
7. Coughs
8. Stress
9. Insomnia
10. Lower back pain

Homeopathic medicines for skin problems are:

1. Medoohinum
2. Lithium Carb
3. Caladium
4. Belladonna
5. Astacus Fluv

⚘

Consult your healthcare practitioner.

45. Horsetail

AKA: Equisetum arvense

No other herb in the entire plant kingdom is as rich in silicon as horsetail. Used in both ancient Chinese and Tibetan medicine, horsetail is still used by herbalists all over the world today. Silicon is the material which collagen is made from. Collagen is the 'body glue' that gives the skin its muscular tone and elasticity. Normal regeneration of healthy tissues in the skin requires silicon.

Horsetail has been used to improve the strength, tone, and texture of the skin, hair and nails. This herb may also be used to relieve itching, irritation and inflammation associated with skin conditions such as eczema, whilst also improving circulation and rejuvenating the connective tissue.

Horsetail has been found to be effective in the topical control of allergic contact skin diseases, which may be related to its anti-inflammatory and wound healing properties.

Consult your healthcare practitioner.

46. Hydrocortisione

AKA: Corticosteroid

Prescription steroid creams and ointments may be recommended for controlling mild to moderate atopic dermatitis. These are available in a variety of strengths, with the least potent one available without a prescription being hydrocortisone 1 per cent cream. Other stronger ointments require a prescription. While stronger oral steroids like prednisone are occasionally used to treat severe eczema, they are not recommended for frequent use due to their side effects.

Hydrocortisone is similar to a natural hormone produced by your adrenal glands and is often used when your body does not make enough of it. Used to treat a multitude of problems including skin ailments, hydrocortisone is known to relieve inflammation and reduce swelling, as well as minimise the itching and redness of conditions like eczema.

Short courses (less than four weeks) of hydrocortisone are usually safe and do not cause any problems. If used for long periods of time, topical steroids can thin your skin, or produce permanent stretchmarks. They may also result in allergic contact dermatitis, acne (particularly if used regularly on the face and around the mouth), rosacea, hair growth in the site of the application and small spots on the body around the hair follicles, known as folliculitis.

While early skin thinning can be reversible if the steroid is stopped, extended use of the topical steroid can cause irreversible stretch marks to develop on the skin. When using the steroid cream, extra care must be taken when applying it on the eyelid area. Generally, it is best to use mild steroids for a maximum of seven days at a time. If eczema on the eyelid remains a problem, it is certainly recommended to see a doctor to discuss alternative treatments.

Some topical steroid creams can also travel through the skin and into the bloodstream. However the amount that reaches the bloodstream is often small and usually causes no problems, unless strong topical steroids are used on a regular basis and on large areas of skin. Children who need frequent courses of strong topical steroids are a concern because the steroid can have an effect on their growth. These children should have their growth monitored.

Yet despite these necessary precautions, it is also possible to be too cautious of steroids. Parents with an unfounded fear of topical steroids may end up under-treating their children's eczema. They may not apply the steroid as often as prescribed or at the strength needed to clear up the breakout. Conversely, this may actually lead to using more steroid cream in the long-term, as the inflamed skin may never completely clear. Results from a study show that a short burst of a potent steroid is as effective and safe as prolonged use of a weak preparation for mild or moderate atopic eczema.

Although side effects from using a mild topical steroid like hydrocortisone occur only rarely, you can reduce the risk further by applying the preparation thinly to the affected areas only no more than twice a day, or as directed by your healthcare practitioner.

Consult your healthcare practitioner.

47. Hypnotherapy

Hypnosis communicates directly with the unconscious mind, which controls many of the processes that influence the immune system. As result, neuro-linguistic programming (NLP) and hypnotherapy used as treatments for skin conditions can help to alleviate the symptoms of psoriasis, eczema and itching.

Skin conditions that cause itching are all affected by stress, depression and other emotions. Using NLP and hypnotherapy, it is possible to learn how to 'switch off' certain sensations.

Have you ever noticed that when you perform a stressful or exciting activity, you start to itch more? One of the reasons stress causes itchy skin is because it releases neuropeptides, molecules that nerve cells use to communicate with each other. They are also involved in causing inflammatory responses in your skin, which you feel as an itch.

Hypnosis is an ideal method of breaking this itchy and vicious cycle because it works on improving emotional states and utilising subconscious processes to promote healthy skin function, and in doing so, reduce the itch.

As a natural treatment, hypnotherapy aims to use the innate healing power of one's own mind and body. Hypnosis is well known to be useful in controlling pain and sometimes this proves useful in reducing the urge to scratch, even relieving itches and scratches experienced at night.

Hypnotherapy may help with these common problems that may make you itch:

1. Nervousness
2. Fear
3. Anxiety
4. Stress
5. Insomnia
6. Frustration
7. Anger
8. Depression

Consult your healthcare practitioner.

48. Immunosuppressants

Eczema is not fully understood and appears to be composed of multiple sub-types that may be distinct diseases. One common thread however, is that the immune system is causing inflammation in the skin which leads to itching, redness, and a skin breakdown that is common to all forms of eczema. Drugs that weaken the immune system may be recommended for people with severe eczema who do not improve with other treatments. Treatment with these drugs can cause serious side effects, including an increased risk of infection.

There are a number of immunosuppressants, but the three most commonly used for treating eczema are cyclosporine, methotrexate, and mycophenolate. Most doctors and patients would prefer to avoid these medications at all costs, but in severe cases the risk-benefit ratio may warrant their consideration.

Consult your healthcare practitioner.

49. Iron

Iron deficiency is the most common cause of anaemia worldwide, primarily due to poor diet among those living in poverty. It is also a factor in many skin conditions.

The signs and symptoms of iron deficiency depend on whether the patient is anaemic, and if so, how fast the anaemia develops. Often there are changes to the hair, skin, nails and mucous membranes. In some patients itching may be present, creating a 'crawling' sensation. Low iron levels can also cause itchy scalp, especially in women.

One way to alleviate the low iron problem is to start consuming dark green vegetables. These can be consumed as a smoothie in the morning or in a salad at lunch or dinnertime.

Consult your healthcare practitioner.

50. Jewelweed–Pale and Spotted

AKA: *Impatiens pallida, Impatiens biflora, touch-me-not*

The Native Americans were the first to use jewelweed as an anti-inflammatory and for its many other medicinal purposes. Numerous tribes used the plant to heal poison ivy rashes, nettle stings, itchy hives, burns and diseases such as measles.

Although the general public trusts the healing properties of jewelweed, the scientific community place little, if any, medicinal value on the plant. Many consider the plant a weed and its curative properties an old wives' tale or folk remedy.

The jewelweed plant contains several chemicals thought to have strong anti-inflammatory and even antifungicidal properties. The leaves and roots contain a chemical called lawsone, which has both anti-inflammatory and antihistamine properties. Other compounds found in the plant called balsaminones have strong anti-itching properties. Jewelweed seed has also been found to contain several potent antimicrobial proteins and anti-carcinogenic compounds.

All of these chemicals combined can be an effective treatment for itching and any kind of irritation, especially those associated with bee stings, nettle, cuts, acne, mosquito bites, burns, and athlete's foot.

The best way to use jewelweed is to break off the stem, crush it, and then rub the juice on the affected area. The juice can also be combined with water and turned into frozen ice cubes to use on itchy spots. Poultices and salves from jewelweed also help to relieve itching and can be used year round for various skin irritations.

Jewelweed Anti-Itch Salve

You will need:

4 cups of freshly washed jewelweed, coarsely chopped

2 cups of olive or coconut oil

1½ - 2 cups of beeswax

2 drops of kunzea

2 drops of lavender

10 drops of sweet orange oil

Method:

1. Bring to boil and simmer jewelweed and olive oil for an hour.
2. Infuse the mixture by letting the mixture sit for 8 hours overnight.
3. Strain the mixture. Clean the pot for further use.
4. Add beeswax into the clean pot and add infused oil.

5. Check the consistency of the mixture by dropping a little bit onto a spoon and place in the freezer. If the mixture is too thin, add more beeswax.
6. Add essential oils.
7. Pour into a glass jar for storage.

A combination of soothing essential oils like chamomile, calendula, benzoin or cedarwood can be used in the Jewelweed Anti-Itch Salve.

Tea tree could replace kunzea oil.

Consult your healthcare practitioner.

51. Jojoba Oil

AKA: Simmondsia sinensis

Jojoba oil is extracted from seeds found in the jojoba bush, which originates from the Sonoran Desert. Centuries ago early Spanish explorers and missionaries recorded that Native Americans extracted the oil from jojoba seeds to treat sores and wounds. They believed the mystical powers of jojoba would alleviate myriad bodily ills and cure external ailments such as cuts, scratches and open sores.

Although jojoba is seen as oil, it is actually liquid wax. In fact, its molecular structure is very similar to that of sebum, the natural oil produced by the skin, which means that it absorbs very easily and does not feel greasy.

This compatibility with our skin's natural oil makes it unique among other oils – jojoba naturally replenishes lost moisture that can cause dryness and itching. Its therapeutic properties mean it can be used for both dry skin and eczema. Only one application is needed throughout the day.

Consult your healthcare practitioner.

52. Juniper

AKA: Juniperus communis

The Greeks recorded using juniper berries as a medicine and the berries have been found in many Egyptian tomb sites including that of Tutankhamun. The Romans used juniper as a cheap domestically-produced substitute for imported Indian black pepper.

Juniper was one of the plants used during the Black Plague to cleanse the house and to bless and protect its inhabitants. Ancient Native Americans also used juniper to cure itches.

Juniper has antiseptic, antimicrobial and anti-inflammatory properties. The tree's therapeutic oil comes from the berries. The resins and tars contained in the oil can also be used to benefit psoriasis sufferers.

To extract the essential oil from the dried ripe berries, a steam distillation process is used. This aromatic oil has a light, fruity fragrance that can be applied topically to ease itchy, eczema prone skin.

An essential oil extracted from juniper berries is used in aromatherapy and perfumery. The essential oil can be distilled out of the berries which have already been used for making gin.

⚓

Juniper and Clove Balm

You will need:

6 tablespoons of coconut oil

2 tablespoons of beeswax

5 tablespoons of juniper berries

3 tablespoons of ground cloves

Method:

1. Melt the coconut oil and beeswax in separate saucepans.
2. Carefully pour and blend them together.
3. Add the juniper berries and cloves.
4. Stir well and let cool.
5. Strain through a muslin cloth.
6. Pour into a glass jar for storage.

⚓

Consult your healthcare practitioner.

53. Kukui Nut Oil

AKA: *Aleurites moluccanus*

The history of the kukui nut shows that early Polynesian settlers brought the tree to the Hawaiian Islands. Also known as the 'candlenut,' the kukui nut tree is found all over the tropics but is mostly seen in Polynesia and Hawaii.

Hawaiians have been using kukui nut oil for hundreds of years to protect and heal skin exposed to the elements. It has a high concentration of essential fatty acids (EFA) that are vital for healthy, vibrant skin. It is a rich source of vitamin A, C and E – all of which offer many benefits for the skin.

Kukui nut oil is easily absorbed into the skin, helping to relieve eczema and dry skin.

Consult your healthcare practitioner.

54. Kunzea

AKA: Kunzea Ambigua

Kunzea oil was used by native Aborigines to relieve red, dry and irritated skin. Derived from the branches of Kunzea Ambigua in north-east Tasmania, the bushes of the plant are topped mechanically. Green matter is then steam distilled to extract the essential oil.

Kunzea essential oil has a unique composition, with a high content of important sesquiterpene compounds. These chemical compounds are important for curbing and moderating inflammatory reactions in the body. In other oils, these molecules may exist separately or at most, in threes. In kunzea oil however, all five of the molecules needed to repair the skin are present.

Kunzea oil has had positive results in the treatment of rashes, skin irritations, eczema and acne. It has been found to be non-irritating and generally well tolerated by users. The Australian Therapeutic Goods Administration has listed kunzea oil for external skin application.

Consult your healthcare practitioner.

55. Lavender

AKA: *Lavandula angustifolia*

Derived from the Latin word 'lavare', which translates to 'wash', lavender is one of the most versatile botanical extracts available for skincare. Used by the Romans to bath and cleanse wounds, lavender is antibacterial, anti-inflammatory, antifungal and practically anti-everything. Lavender is thought to stimulate cellular growth and regeneration in the skin by helping your upper layer of skin rejuvenate itself. The fact that lavender calms down inflammation, speeds up wound healing and deals with infection means it has a beneficial effect on eczema. It is one of the only essential oils that is safe to use directly on the skin.

It is considered by some to be the quintessential English garden herb and was highly regarded in the Victorian times for its classic fragrance in fancy soaps, sachets, potpourris and perfumes; healing properties; use as a household cleanser; a culinary ingredient; and a disinfectant.

Lavender is also important as a medicinal herb. Lavender contains compounds that bind to the same receptors as the valium family of tranquilizers, suggesting that the herb has the same effect. It also helps to boost the immune system.

⚘

Lavender and Calendula Anti-Itch Salve

You will need:

40ml of olive oil

30g of beeswax

2 vitamin E capsules

10 drops of lavender essential oil

10 drops of calendula oil

Method:

1. Combine all the ingredients in a bowl.
2. Place the bowl over a saucepan of hot water.
3. Puncture the vitamin E capsules and blend together.
4. Let cool slightly and pour into a small jar or balm tin.

⚘

Consult your healthcare practitioner.

56. Liquorice

AKA: Glycyrrhiza glabra

In Europe liquorice has been considered a valued medicine and a trade commodity for at least a thousand years. In China it is still used in more applications than any other herb – even more than ginseng. Not just a tasty sweet, liquorice is actually a great leafy plant from which the root is harvested for use in food and herbal medicine.

Liquorice contains a compound called glycyrrhizin, which has been shown to have anti-inflammatory activity. In 2003 a clinical trial was undertaken to look at the effects of applying a liquorice gel to people with dermatitis. After two weeks, redness, swelling and itching had decreased significantly in the 100+ people studied as part of the trial. The study also found that liquorice extract could be considered an effective herb in the treatment of eczema.

Liquorice Oil Infusion

You will need:

liquorice root

olive oil

Method:

To make a simple oil infusion, chop a liquorice root and combine with olive oil. Put the root into a glass jar and cover it with enough oil to leave a half-inch layer of liquid above the herb. Screw the lid on tightly and put it in a warm place, preferably not in sunlight. Leave for one month. After a month strain the oil through muslin cloth, bottle and keep refrigerated.

The infusion can be added with one cup of finely ground oatmeal to a tepid bath to help relieve itching.

Apply the cool oil to itchy skin as necessary.

Consult your healthcare practitioner.

57. Magnesium

AKA: Mg

Magnesium is everywhere in the body and is the fourth most abundant mineral. Responsible for hundreds of different biochemical reactions and enzyme systems, it supports important processes like protein synthesis, cell growth and energy production. It even has roles in nerve function, muscle control and blood pressure, with blood sugar regulation depending on magnesium.

It is no surprise then that magnesium oil is considered the gold standard for rapidly restoring cellular magnesium through the skin. And for those who can tolerate it, magnesium and other detoxing baths can be helpful in healing the skin.

A concentrated transdermal magnesium supplement, absorbable magnesium oil contains only raw, ultra-pure magnesium chloride and other trace minerals. Although this helps condition the skin and energize the body, some people cannot tolerate magnesium. In some cases, it can actually cause a prickly feeling on the skin.

Magnesium oil blended with plant butters and oils can be tolerated when applied to the skin. These creams can add hydration and help in normalising the skin barrier, providing emollient protection, as well as the opportunity to absorb nutrients like magnesium.

Taking a magnesium supplement internally will also help with an itch problem.

ॐ

10 Benefits of Using Magnesium

1. Essential for muscle and nerve function
2. Converts blood sugar into energy
3. Helps to relieve stress
4. Aids in fighting depression
5. Promotes healthier cardiovascular system
6. Keeps teeth healthy
7. Prevents calcium deposits, kidney and gallstones
8. Relieves indigestion
9. Helps with muscle recovery
10. Balances electrolytes

ॐ

Consult your healthcare practitioner.

58. Marshmallow

AKA: *Althea officinalis*

The traditional medicinal uses of marshmallow are reflected in the plant's biological family name, which comes from the Greek word *althainein,* meaning 'to heal.' Greek physician Hippocrates described the value of althea in the treatment of wounds. The Romans, Chinese, Egyptians and Syrians used marshmallow as a source of food, while the Arabs made poultices from its leaves and applied them to the skin to reduce inflammation.

This plant is a very useful medicinal herb as its soothing properties make it very effective in treating inflammation and irritations of the skin, particularly when it comes to eczema. The whole plant (in particular the root) is high in mucilage, a gel-like substance that is an effective emollient.

For a simple remedy to relieve itching skin, take some powdered marshmallow root and add some water. Mix it well and apply to the affected area. Leave for a few minutes and then clean off the mixture with a soft cloth.

Consult your healthcare practitioner.

59. Milk Thistle

AKA: Silybum marianum

Milk thistle, which also goes by the names of bull thistle, holy thistle, royal thistle and prickly thistle, is a plant that has been used medicinally for over 2000 years.

Commonly found growing wild on roadsides, along fence lines and in pastures, this herb is native to the Mediterranean, although it now grows wild all over the world. Considered an invasive weed in some areas, milk thistle seeds have antioxidant properties that are many times stronger than vitamin E. Given its name for its milky sap, milk thistle sap is a demulcent – meaning it creates a gel-like layer, trapping moisture and soothing the skin.

Milk thistle contains silymarin, a compound that was the subject of a study by Italian researchers in 2008. In the study, a product that contained milk thistle was given to a group of people suffering from rosacea to use over a month's period. The results showed an overall improvement in redness, itchiness, hydration and skin colour. Other anecdotal evidence confirms the study's finding, showing milk thistle to alleviate the symptoms of eczema.

Milk thistle is also an extremely powerful liver protector and enhancer. Your liver is charged with clearing various substances through your body, meaning liver integrity is essential to your overall health and longevity. This is even truer for eczema sufferers, whose livers work overtime, trying to clear certain substances. Taking a dose of milk thistle or drinking milk thistle tea may help reduce your eczema symptoms.

Take a cup of tea three times daily using 1 teaspoon of milkthistle seeds infused for 10 to 15 minutes in boiling water. Alternatively, 40 drops of tincture in water may be taken three times daily.

Milk thistle is remarkably safe. It has rated in all the great herbal guides as a cure for many diseases. It causes no side effects in most people who use it, though a few people have reported mild stomach upset or slight reactions.

Consult your healthcare practitioner.

60. Minerals

Eye, hair, nails, mouth and skin symptoms are among the early outward signs of a vitamin and mineral deficiency. Minerals are essential in the breakdown of food during digestion, and some are instrumental in maintaining fluid balance inside cells. Those that are currently considered essential for human nutrition are calcium, phosphorus, iron, potassium, selenium, magnesium and zinc.

Many more minerals, however, are needed to maintain optimal health. Chromium, cobalt, copper, manganese and potassium are thought to be equally as important. A mineral deficiency, especially magnesium, may present itself as itchy skin.

Consult your healthcare practitioner.

61. Mugwort

AKA: Artemisia douglasiana

Mugwort has a long history of use in folk medicine. Anglo-Saxon tribes were particularly fond of using the aromatic mugwort, believing it to be one of the nine sacred herbs given to the world by the god Woden.

A member of the daisy family, mugwort is a hardy plant that is drought tolerant and nearly impossible to kill. Also a topical anaesthetic, mugwort has both antibacterial and antifungal properties.

Fresh, crushed mugwort leaves applied to the skin can relieve burning, itching and pain. With continued application, this herb can also be used to remove warts.

To treat itchy skin, bathe the affected area in mugwort tea – simply boil fresh leaves and apply to the problem area.

Consult your healthcare practitioner.

62. Myrrh

AKA: Commiphora myrrha

According to Chinese medicine, a healthy body is dependent on blood movement. In China, myrrh is often used as a blood tonic to improve circulation and bring fresh oxygen and nutrients to the organs and tissues.

Myrrh is taken from Commiphora myrrha trees, which are commonly found in the Arabian Peninsula. It is harvested as dried sap and has a sweet, woody fragrance. The sap has been used for centuries to make medicines designed to decrease inflammation and kill bacteria.

The use of myrrh goes back at least 4,000 years, with historical data showing it is one of the oldest known herbs used for medicinal purposes. In fact, myrrh can even be found in an Ancient Egyptian list of over 800 prescriptions and recipes.

Myrrh is harvested from the stems of bushy shrubs that grow in Arabia, Somalia, and other parts of North Africa and the Middle East. Both an immune and circulatory stimulant, myrrh is also an expectorant, a medicine that helps heals coughs. Taken internally and externally, it can be used to heal infections, repair wounds and remove poisons from the body.

A common ingredient in many skin care products today, myrrh is known for promoting healthy skin as it prevents the signs of aging and soothes racked, chapped skin. Suitable for treating chronic wounds and ulcers, this ancient plant is known to accelerate healing and is especially effective in the treatment of weeping eczema. It can be used in cold compresses to relieve both sores and wounds.

Add it to creams and lotions to help relieve skin infections like athlete's foot, ringworm, weeping eczema, bedsores, boils carbuncles, itching and acne.

Myrrh and Frankincense Balm

You will need:

¼ cup of olive oil

¼ cup of coconut oil

¼ cup of shea nut butter

6 vitamin E capsules

10 drops of myrrh oil

10 drops of frankincense oil

Method:

1. Combine the ingredients in a bowl.
2. Place the bowl over a saucepan of hot water.
3. Blend together and let cool slightly.
4. Pour into balm tins before the mixture sets.

Consult your healthcare practitioner.

63. Neem

AKA: *Azardica indica*

The leaves of the neem tree have long been used in the traditional Hindu medicine Ayurveda. Used in Indian medicine for over 4,000 years, neem is an anti-inflammatory that can reduce redness and irritation, thanks to the two main anti-inflammatory substances found in the leaves, nimbin and nimbidin. Impressively, these substances have been shown to have anti-inflammatory properties comparable to common non-steroids and steroidal drugs.

Because it relieves pain, some people report instant relief from the excruciating discomfort of eczema as soon as they apply neem salve or cream. Also containing anti-bacterial properties, neem can be used to clean up secondary infections and better yet, it can prevent them from happening in the first place.

In addition to moisturising the skin, neem can achieve most of what steroid creams, antibiotics and antihistamines do, without the side effects.

Research suggests neem may be just as effective as over-the-counter and prescription eczema medication. Needless to say, Indian people agree.

Consult your healthcare practitioner.

64. Oats

AKA: *Avena sativa*

For thousands of years oatmeal has been used to soothe and relieve various skin conditions and inflammations. This soothing plant has a history of being used in baths to cure itchy skin.

Although whole oat flour provides effective topical relief, the use of standardized oat extracts will help achieve clinical benefits due to their remarkable chemical composition. Some studies have shown that the avenanthramides (a group of micronutrients) and the 20 or so phenols (chemical compounds) found in oatmeal help reduce inflammation caused by the allergens that irritate skin. These phenols have also been shown to have high antioxidant activity.

Avenanthramides are only found in oats and are able to inhibit the release of the inflammatory cytokines (small proteins) that are present in many itchy skin conditions like eczema and dermatitis. Oat kernel extracts with standardized levels of avenanthramides are often used in skin, hair, baby and sun care products.

Itchy, dry skin often has a high pH level which oatmeal helps to normalize. Providing relief from eczema symptoms, this can also help to break the 'itch and scratch' cycle. Additionally, saponins (chemical components found in oatmeal), allow the grain to function as an effective natural cleanser. Oatmeal is also believed to have antifungal properties.

Many laboratories continue to conduct studies on this interesting grain.

$\wp$

Oatmilk Bath

You will need:

Muslin cloth

Finely ground oatmeal

Lavender oil

Chamomile oil

Method:

1. Tie the finely ground oatmeal into a muslin cloth.
2. Place under running water. The colloidal activity of the fine ground oatmeal should make the water milky.
3. Add a couple of drops of lavender and chamomile to your bathwater.
4. Use the muslin cloth as your washcloth.

You could also add calendula oil or chamomile oil to the bath.

$\wp$

Consult your healthcare practitioner.

65. Opiates

AKA: Laudanum, Cocaine, Opium

Today it is hard to believe that in early and mid-Victorian Britain it was possible to walk into a chemist and by cocaine, laudanum and even arsenic. Opium preparations were even sold freely in the market stalls of towns and in the countryside by travelling hawkers.

Paracelsus, a 16th century Swiss-German alchemist, discovered that the alkaloids in opium are far more soluble in alcohol than water. He made a specific tincture of opium that was of considerable use in controlling pain. The tincture, which he named laudanum, was a combination of opium, alcohol, crushed pearls, musk, amber and other additives. Laudanum was used in many medicines to relieve pain, to produce sleep and to allay irritation.

Opiates including morphine and codeine are currently used in modern medicine for pain relief, but are not recommended for treating skin conditions.

Consult your healthcare practitioner.

66. Oregon Grape Root

AKA: Mahonia aquifolium

O regon grape root is a tall, flowering shrub that grows in abundance in the Pacific Northwest region of the United States. While it is not botanically related to the endangered goldenseal, both plants contain the immune-stimulating, infection-fighting and antiseptic constituent berberine. As a result, herbalists sometimes substitute Oregon grape root for goldenseal or the Chinese herb, coptis. The plant's root and root-like stem are used for making medicine.

'Dermatologic Therapy' published a clinical study in 2010 designed to discern which plant extracts and compounds worked best for a variety of skin diseases. Of the various skin diseases tested, atopic eczema and psoriasis showed the most impressive results with Oregon grape root treatment.

Previously used as a remedy for constipation, bloating and other intestinal issues, dermatologists are now studying the plant's effectiveness in treating psoriasis, eczema and other skin diseases. An Oregon grape wash can be used to deter the over production of plaque cells that occur in people who suffer from skin conditions like psoriasis.

Consult your healthcare practitioner.

67. Parsley

AKA: *Petroselinum crispum*

Revered by the Ancient Greeks and mentioned by the Romans as early as the fourth century BC, parsley has a long and romantic history.

And it isn't just useful for its taste and smell – rich in nutrients, parsley has a number of medicinal properties. Ounce for ounce, parsley contains more essential vitamins than any other herb. It helps with skin irritations and itchiness, digestion, gout, halitosis and kidney ailments.

Additionally, parsley has the ability to inhibit histamines in the body, meaning it can decrease the symptoms of allergies and inflammatory responses like eczema flare-ups. Roots, leaves and seeds can all be used to treat your itch.

Consult your healthcare practitioner.

68. Patchouli

AKA: Pogostemon cablin

Patchouli is native to India and Malaysia. Traditionally, leaves from the patchouli plant were placed between Indian cashmere shawls on route to Victorian England to protect the merchandise from moths (without this signature scent of dried patchouli leaves, the shawls could not be sold in England).

Although this essential oil may remind people of the hippie era because of its use in incense sticks, its value in skin care is incalculable. Patchouli oil improves with age, meaning older oils can be more expensive than the newer ones. The therapeutic properties of patchouli are antiseptic, astringent, deodorant, fungicide, insecticide, sedative and tonic.

When applied to the skin the oil is one of the most active tissue regenerators and helps to stimulate the growth of new skin cells. In wounds, it not only promotes faster healing, but also prevents scarring when the wound heals. It can be used to improve dry itchy scalp conditions and get rid of dandruff.

Patchouli oil is very effective in soothing rough, cracked and overly dehydrated skin. It is used to treat acne, eczema, sores, ulcers, fungal infections and scalp disorders.

~

Patchouli Scented Balm

You will need:

40ml of coconut oil

30g of beeswax

4 vitamin E capsules

8 drops of bergamot oil

8 drops of orange oil

4 drops of patchouli oil

Method:

1. Combine the ingredients in a bowl.
2. Place the bowl over a saucepan of hot water.
3. Pierce the capsules and add the vitamin E oil.
4. Blend together and let cool slightly.
5. Pour into small balm tins for storage.

~

Consult your healthcare practitioner.

69. Pawpaw

AKA: *Carica papaya*

Christopher Columbus called it the 'fruit of angels' but Australians and New Zealanders prefer to call it pawpaw. Originally found in tropical American countries, today Carica papaya is cultivated in most topical countries around the world. It was first studied over 100 years ago by a man named Dr Lucas, who transformed the fermented fruit of the tree into an ointment still used today.

One benefit pawpaw ointments have over other eczema creams is that they come from a natural source without added fragrances or dyes. Additives in creams may dry out or irritate the skin, thus aggravating the eczema. Pawpaw contains many nutrients including vitamin C, folate, fibre, vitamin A, magnesium, potassium, copper, and pantothenic acid.

Pawpaw ointments can be used to moisturise the skin but may not be potent enough to relieve everybody's itching.

Consult your healthcare practitioner.

70. Peach Kernel Oil

AKA: *Prunus persica*

Historically, Romans were the first to recognise the beneficial properties of peach kernel oil. Purchased directly from Persia during the reign of the Emperor Claudius, peach kernel oil was a prized beauty treatment in Ancient Rome. It wasn't until the first half of the sixteenth century that this useful oil became popular in England. It has been used for skincare ever since.

Peach kernel oil is extracted from the kernel of the peach and is rich in polyunsaturated fatty acids including oleic acid and linoleic acid, which helps the skin lock in moisture and retain elasticity. Due to its special molecular structure, it penetrates easily into the cells.

Much like almond and apricot kernel oils, peach kernel oil is suitable for dry and sensitive skin and is useful for relieving itching. It absorbs easily but slowly. A mild oil, peach kernel can be used on most skin types.

Consult your healthcare practitioner.

71. Perilla Seed Oil

AKA: Perilla fructescens

The perilla plant has a long history of use in traditional Chinese medicine for a wide variety of ailments. Historically, Perilla was used to treat stomach ache, coughs, asthma and as an antibacterial.

Obtained from the seeds of the perilla herb, perilla seed oil is a rich source of unsaturated fatty acids, vitamins and amino acids. It is frequently used in cooking and is also used along with synthetic resins in the production of varnishes. Still, it is best known for its cosmetic properties and can be used to treat dry and itchy skin.

This member of the mint family is also called:

Wild coleus

Chinese basil

Shiso

Purple mint

Rattlesnake weed.

Consult your healthcare practitioner.

72. Phosphorus

Phosphorus is an essential mineral found most commonly in the body as phosphate. While it is required for healthy cell function and is a major component of bone, high levels of phosphorus in the body, known as hyperphosphatemia, can lead to chronic itching.

The best way to reduce phosphorus in your blood and itching on your skin is to maintain a low phosphorus diet. You can also reduce phosphorus by taking a phosphorus binder that absorbs phosphorus in the gut before it enters your blood.

Additionally, taking the active form of vitamin D will help balance calcium and phosphorus levels. Taking calcimimetic medicine can also potentially lower phosphorus and keep your bones healthy.

Reduce Foods High in Phosphorus

Foods high in phosphorus include:

cheese

ice cream

milk

yoghurt

processed meats

organ meats

sardines

brown and wild rice

bran products

whole grain products

dried beans and peas

beer

chocolate drinks

Cola type beverages

chocolate

nuts

nut butters and spreads

seeds.

Consult your healthcare practitioner.

73. Plantain

AKA: Plantago major, ripple grass, white man's foot

Used by ancient tribes to heal the bites of insects and ease the sting of nettle and poison ivy, plantain leaves have been used by cultures all over the world. Considered by the Saxons to be one of the nine sacred herbs, legend has it that Alexander the Great discovered plantain and brought it back to Europe in 327 BC. Humble and hardy, plantain is a mainstay of traditional European and American herbalism.

A 'contact healer,' crushed plantain leaves can be applied to bites, stings and other skin irritations for quick relief. In addition, plantain is also effective when used on psoriasis, eczema and rashes.

Containing high levels of vitamin A, vitamin C and calcium, plantain is also jam-packed with beneficial chemicals including allantion, apigenin, aucubin, baicalein, linoleic acid, oleanolic acid, sorbitol and tannin. Like many herbal folk remedies, the plant has high antibacterial, antimicrobial and anti-inflammatory qualities. Considered one of the world's best herbs for treating wounds, researchers are currently studying its effects on lowering blood sugar levels.

The seed husks from Plantago psyllium are sold under the international brand name Metamucil. These wild seeds are rich in omega-3 fatty acids, which may help relieve the itch of eczema when incorporated into your diet.

Plantain leaves can be used as food, with the plant's young leaves making a great addition to salads. It may also be used as tincture, wash, balm, or tea. The recipe below is a natural energy and immune booster, packed full of antioxidants. A great internal cleanser, this super-charged smoothie makes for a healthy, fast breakfast.

Plantain Medicinal Green Juice

You will need:

A small handful of plantain and kale

A small handful of grapes

1 kiwifruit

1 granny smith apple

1 celery stalk

250ml of coconut water

Method:

Use a blender or a juicer to combine all of the above ingredients into a superfood smoothie or juice.

If desired, you may also add nuts or seeds to the recipe.

Consult your healthcare practitioner.

74. Probiotics

Probiotics are important in maintaining a healthy bowel and skin. Lactobacillus is a type of friendly bacteria that lives in the digestive, urinary and genital systems without causing disease. There are many different species of lactobacillus, some of which can be found in fermented foods like yoghurt and in dietary supplements. Lactobacillus can be used for skin disorders such as fever blisters, canker sores, eczema and acne.

Taking a strong probiotic supplement daily that contains bifidus and lactobacillus may boost the immune system and control allergy symptoms.

It is thought that giving a baby probiotics helps to stave off eczema and other allergic diseases by beneficially altering the early colonisation of bacteria in their gut, which may help the baby's immune system develop and mature.

Consult your healthcare practitioner.

75. Purslane

AKA: *Portulaca oleracea*

While it may be considered more of a weed and less of an herb, purslane has many useful qualities that can be used to help eczema. Also known as verdolaga, pigweed, little hogweed, pusley, and pourpier, purslane is found on every populated continent and is one of the eight most common plants in the world.

Despite being the subject of many studies, purslane's benefits are still relatively unknown to the average individual. Rich in vitamins and minerals, it is unfortunate the wide range of nutritional and medicinal benefits of purslane are not conventional knowledge.

Packed with vitamin A, B, C, and E, as well as iron, calcium, magnesium, potassium, folate and lithium, purslane also has the highest level of omega-3 essential fatty acids, helpful against inflammation, of all land-based vegetables. All of these vitamins and minerals make purslane an effective tool for treating eczema.

Consult your healthcare practitioner.

76. Red Clover

AKA: Trifolium pratense

Although red clover originates from Central Europe, it has spread to most corners of the world thanks to the simple conditions in which it grows. For this reason, the plant has been used in medicine by many cultures throughout history.

Red clover is rich in isoflavones, oestrogen-like substances, and its use in medicine goes back centuries, with a history of both topical and internal applications. As a topical aid, red clover is often an ingredient in liniments and balms used for relieving the pain of both eczema and psoriasis. It is also found in treatments for sores and burns, and aids against skin cancer.

The pain relieving properties of red clover are due to the presence of the anti-inflammatory compounds eugenol, myricetin and the salicylic acid in the flowers. While salicylic acid is known to fight eczema, red clover can be used to treat an array of other skin conditions because it contains essential vitamins for the skin such as vitamin A and vitamin B complex. Red clover oil is also rich in iron.

Red clover oil comes from the plant's blossom and is widely used to treat eczema in both adults and children. Because of its ability to promote healthy skin, red clover oil may be used in massages. It has calcium and magnesium which tones and relaxes the nervous system, relieving tension caused by stress and anxiety. By reducing stress levels the oil may help break the itch-scratch cycle. Red clover oil may also be combined with other purifying herbs such as burdock.

Red Clover can be used for these skin problems:

- sores
- burns
- itching
- eczema
- psoriasis
- acne
- canker sores
- veins.

Eczema Tea

You will need:

1 part chickweed

1 part red clover

1 part nettle

Method:

Rub the dried herbs until they resemble tea leaves. Store in a glass jar and use 1 teaspoon to 1 cup of boiling water.

Consult your healthcare practitioner.

77. Rice Bran

AKA: Oryza Sativa

Well known in Asia for its health benefits, traditionally Japanese women would rub rice bran on their faces to keep their skin smooth and bright.

For eczema sufferers, the outer layer of the grain, or the rice bran, can be directly applied to the skin and used as an exfoliant. This ancient grain works in much the same way as oatmeal does when easing itchy skin.

While the nutritional value of rice is well known, less obvious are the medicinal and cosmetic applications of rice bran. Rice seeds and bran have been used for thousands of years to relieve inflammation associated with skin diseases, and for cleansing and softening the skin.

Consult your healthcare practitioner.

78. Rosehip Oil

AKA: Rosa canina

Rosehip oil may have been the first plant distilled by the Arabs. Commercially cultivated by the people of Persia, Greece and Rome in the 16th century, rosehip oil also has a long history of use in traditional Chinese medicine. More recently rosehip was given to soldiers during the First World War, due to the shortage of citrus fruit.

Rosehip oil extract is obtained by cold pressing rosehip seeds. This oil has a high content of vitamin A and vitamin C, making it ideal for use on the skin. Rosehip oil is also packed with healthy fatty acids, including linolenic, myristic, palmitic, stearic, oleic, arachidic, gadoleic, eicosenoic, behenic and palmitoleic acids.

As a result, rosehip oil can be used to improve many skin ailments. Particularly suited to dry, mature skin, this oil can help constrict the capillaries to reduce the appearance of thread veins and speed up the cellular activity of the skin.

Its tonic and soothing qualities are also helpful in reducing inflammation and irritation. Absorbing quickly into the skin, rosehip oil is frequently used in cosmetics and is a great natural source of retinoic acid, which helps heal eczema, burns and scars.

10 Uses for Rosehips:

1. Rosehip tea
2. Rosehip oil hair conditioner
3. Rosehip jelly
4. Rosehip syrup
5. Rosehip oil nail treatment
6. Rosehip infused vinegar
7. Rosehip wine
8. Rosehip oil moisturiser
9. Rosehip marmalade
10. Rosehip face mask

Consult your healthcare practitioner.

79. Rosemary

AKA: Rosmarinus officinalis

In Ancient Egypt, rosemary was seen as a symbol of regeneration and a way to drive out evil spirits. Today, traces of the plant can still be found in tombs.

While it may or may not be able to remove evil spirits, rosemary has many other proven benefits. An effective antiseptic, rosemary oil is also known for its antibacterial and antifungal qualities.

Rosemary oil is also a great antioxidant and is considered to be one of the strongest ones available in nature. Subsequently, it is widely used in the food industry for this purpose.

A well-known herb for the hair, rosemary can be used to treat dandruff and encourage hair regrowth. A few drops of rosemary oil blended with a carrier oil can help ease dry, itchy skin.

❦

Rosemary Scalp Tonic

You will need:

A small spray bottle

1 cup of water

A handful of dried rosemary

3 drops of lavender oil

3 drops of tea tree oil

Method:

1. Boil a cup of water and tip over the dried rosemary.
2. Cover and allow to steep for approximately 15 to 20 minutes.
3. Strain and allow to cool.
4. Once completely cool, pour the rosemary tea into your spray bottle.
5. Add the combined essential oils.

Use the spray tonic on your scalp three or four times a day for the first week and gradually cut back, using it only when you feel the itch returning.

❦

Consult your healthcare practitioner.

80. Rosewood

AKA: *Aniba rosaeodora*

Rosewood oil comes from trees grown in Brazil. Apparently people have used so much rosewood for furniture, flooring, guitars and oils that the tree is now endangered. Today every tree that is cut down must be replaced with another.

Most commonly associated with skin conditions, rosewood oil is known for its regenerating properties that work to repair and replenish skin cells. Acting as a shield for your skin, this oil defends against harmful bacteria, viruses, fungi and other microbes. The natural antiseptic and antibacterial properties found in rosewood make it suitable for treating wounds, cuts, burns and infections, while preventing them from becoming septic. As such, rosewood oil can be used to relieve dry, sensitive, itchy inflamed skin.

Consult your healthcare practitioner.

81. Safflower Oil

AKA: *Carthamus tintorius*

Safflower is native to the Middle East and is widely cultivated throughout Europe and the United States. Although safflower is recognised primarily as a source of healthy edible oil, traditionally this was not the case.

The safflower looks a lot like a thistle and its seeds produce oil that resembles sunflower oil in its makeup. It helps maintain skin elasticity by enabling the skin to retain moisture and by removing dry skin. Used in skin softening cosmetics, safflower oil is also helpful for repairing eczema and dry, rough skin.

Consult your healthcare practitioner.

82. Salicylic Acid

AKA: 2-hydroxybenzoic acid

The first documented use of salicylic acid can be traced all the way back to around 500 BC, when the Ancient Greeks used it primarily as a pain reliever. However, archaeologists have also found traces of the acid in other parts of the world, and in 2014 they successfully identified traces of it on 7th century pottery fragments found in east central Colorado.

Salicylic acid is obtained from the bark of the white willow tree and from the herb meadowsweet. The medicinal part of the plant is the inner bark, which can be used for a variety of ailments. In the 20th century, salicylic acid started to be used as a treatment for skin conditions like acne, psoriasis, warts and calluses.

Because some people are sensitive to salicylic acid, it is recommended to proceed with caution when using it to treat the skin.

Consult your health practitioner.

83. Salt

AKA: Sodium chloride

Salt has been an essential, virtually omnipresent, part of medicine for thousands of years. It has been used in everything from remedies and support treatments to preventative measures.

In Egypt, salt is mentioned as an essential ingredient in some of the country's oldest medical scripts. Both sea salt and rock salt were also well known to the Ancient Greeks who noted that eating salty food affected basic body functions, leading it to be used medically. During the Renaissance a hipbath in salt water was believed to be a superb remedy for skin diseases and itching.

Dead Sea salt is considered to be particularly useful for treating chronic skin diseases such as psoriasis and eczema. This is because the mineral composition of Dead Sea salt is slightly different from that of common sea salt. The Dead Sea in Israel is known for its healing properties and many people with eczema go there to sit in the sun and swim in the water. One clinical study looked at the experience of more than 1,500 people with eczema who had previously stayed at the Dead Sea longer than four weeks, and found that 95 per cent of their skin conditions were cleared. Frequently used in body care products, Dead Sea salt may also be used as an additive to treat eczema.

During the Victorian times people gathered by the seaside to bathe among the waves as they were convinced they would benefit from the practice. It was felt that a quick dip in the salt water would benefit them more than prolonged immersion, because that might bring on a chill and weaken the constitution. Even a brief holiday at the coast would leave people replenished and their skin healthy and glowing. They would return home, speaking with enthusiasm about their coastal holiday.

Salt Therapy Rooms

Salt therapy is a widely used natural remedy dating back to medieval times, when monks acknowledged the healing atmosphere of salt caves. The first salt room was built in Russia and recreated the microclimate of a salt cave.

Sitting in a salt therapy room exposes the body to tiny particles of salt that can cleanse and detoxify the system. The particles enter the upper airway where the salt has the natural ability to absorb and neutralize bacteria and histamines. These particles can have favourable effects on the skin as they kill bacteria and fungi, reducing itching in eczema sufferers.

For best results, make sure the affected skin is directly exposed to the microclimate of the salt room.

Consult your healthcare practitioner.

84. Sandalwood

AKA: Santalum album

S andalwood was used as essential therapeutic oil in both traditional Chinese and Tibetan medicine. A major trade item by 700 BC, sandalwood has even been found in Ancient Egyptian embalming formulations. In China, it is used in incense sticks. Sandalwood is also a major ingredient in many lotions and body oils.

Sandalwood oil is extracted from the wood of the tree. Both the wood and oil produce a distinctive fragrance that has been highly valued for centuries. Recently, sandalwood oil prices have skyrocketed to over $2,000 per kilo of essential oil.

Sandalwood oil is harvested from native trees that are over 30 years old and unfortunately they use all of the tree, from leaves to roots, to obtain the sandalwood oil. The fragrant tree is also at risk from human encroachment due to expanding population and this is impacting on wild tree stocks. Sandalwood is a hemi-parasitic plant, meaning it cannot adequately provide itself the essential nutrients for its growth and sustenance. Often a host plant needs to grow alongside it for support. The future of this highly regarded tree is severely threatened by an increasing demand for Sandalwood.

Many farmers are looking at planting Sandalwood both for its highly valued oil and also to contribute towards reducing salinity and erosion in farming areas. Sandalwood plantations in Western Australia are being financed by private landowners, broadacre farmers, managed investment schemes and government programs.

Sandalwood essential oil helps soften the skin by increasing and restoring its ability to retain moisture. It can be directly applied to the skin and used to relieve localised rashes, inflammation and itching. The cooling and anti-microbial property of sandalwood helps to soothe the skin and heal small abrasions. To reduce itching, a sandalwood paste can be applied to the skin. Also an excellent home remedy for insect bites, sandalwood paste can be used to treat sunburn.

Sandalwood Paste

Mix 3-7 drops of sandalwood essential oil with one teaspoon of turmeric powder and one teaspoon of rose water.

Consult your healthcare practitioner.

85. Sarsaparilla

AKA: Smilax

Sarsaparilla root has been used for centuries by the indigenous people of Central and South America for rheumatism and skin ailments, and as a general tonic for physical weakness. In Peru and Honduras, it has long been used to treat headaches, joint pain and to fight the common cold. Many shamans and medicine men in the Amazon use the sarsaparilla root internally and externally for leprosy and other skin problems, such as psoriasis and dermatitis.

A 1942 study published in the New England Journal of Medicine found sarsaparilla to improve the condition of psoriasis dramatically. The clinical study, which involved 92 patients, showed improved psoriasis lesions in 62 per cent of patients and completely cleared lesions in 18 per cent of patients who used the ingredient to treat their skin condition.

Some of the most fascinating ingredients in sarsaparilla root are saponins, chemical compounds. Saponins, usually bitter to the taste, are named after soap because of the foam-like reactions when they are placed into water. In the plants where they originate, saponin's chemical compounds help deter fungi and insects from eating their leaves. This could be one of the possible reasons that sarsaparilla has anti-fungal properties.

One of the possible causes is sarsaparilla's blood cleansing properties. Individuals with psoriasis have been found to have high levels of endotoxins circulating in the bloodstream. Endotoxins are cell wall fragments of normal gut bacteria. Sarsaponin, one of sarsaparilla's main actives, has been found to bind to these endotoxins and remove them, thus improving psoriasis.

This endotoxin-binding action is probably why the sarsaparilla root has been used for centuries as a blood purifier. Other health conditions associated with high endotoxin levels include eczema, arthritis and ulcerative colitis.

Sarsaparilla can be eaten raw or dried roots can be boiled and taken as tea. It can also be taken as a tincture, in capsule form and as powder.

Consult your healthcare practitioner.

86. Sea Buckthorn

AKA: Hippophae rhammoides

Sea buckthorn is one of the important plants of the mountainous regions of China and Russia. For more than 1,000 years its berries have been used in both Tibetan and Indian medicine practices.

Sea buckthorn oil comes from an infusion of the berries in a vegetable oil. One ingredient in the oil, palmitoleic acid, is also a component found in skin. With high levels of essential fatty acids, sea buckthorn oil is extremely nourishing. More than 40 volatile compounds are also in the fruit and leaves of sea buckthorn, with the oil containing carotenoids, tocopherols, sterols, flavonoids, lipids, ascorbic acid and tannins.

Sea buckthorn is considered a valuable topical agent in treating atopic eczema and the itchy symptoms related to eczema.

Consult your health practitioner.

87. Silver

AKA: Electrically isolated silver

The term 'blue blood' comes from skin discoloration caused by the use of silver cutlery. Long term use of the mineral colloidal silver, a suspension of sub microscopic metallic silver particles in a colloidal base, can lead to the skin turning an ashen grey colour.

Hippocrates, in his writings, discussed the use of silver in wound care and at the beginning of the twentieth century surgeons routinely used silver sutures to reduce the risk of infection. In the early 20th century, physicians used eye drops containing silver to treat ophthalmic problems and various infections. Sometimes, it was even used internally.

Prior to the introduction of modern antibiotics, colloidal silver was used as a germicide and disinfectant. With the development of modern antibiotics in the 1940s, the use of silver as an antimicrobial agent diminished.

Despite this, itchy skin, rashes, hives and allergic reactions can still benefit from the soothing effects of colloidal silver. Topical application of colloidal silver is also recommended for eczema and psoriasis. This is because particles of silver are small enough to penetrate at a cellular level and destroy pathogens of all types, including those that may cause itching, such as bacteria, fungal spores, parasites and viruses.

§

Seven uses for Colloidal Silver Cream or Spray

1. Promote faster healing
2. Stop itching
3. Reduce infection
4. Strengthen immune system
5. Relieve bronchial problems
6. Reduce the effect of cold and flu viruses
7. Eliminate yeast infections

Silver collects in the skin and other organs and does not dissipate. The condition is called argyria. In argyria, silver deposited in the body reacts with the sun through a process similar to that of the development of a photographic negative. This leads to permanent discolouration of the skin. It is estimated that the average person would have to ingest at least two to four grams of silver to develop argyria. To avoid looking like a Smurf or the Tin Man, look at other ways of treating your itch.

§

Consult your healthcare practitioner.

88. Slippery Elm

AKA: Ulmus fulva

The first known people to use the slippery elm tree for medicinal purposes were the Native Americans. They discovered that when the bark of the tree is mixed with water, it transforms into a sticky, glue-like substance. When applied to the skin, this substance dries and becomes a natural bandage. The inner bark is the part of the plant used for medicine.

Native to North America, slippery elm is recognised as one of the best herbs for easing pain and reducing inflammation. Its slippery fibre is very soothing, both internally and externally. Slippery elm contains antioxidants that can boost cell renewal and fight aging.

Consult your healthcare practitioner.

89. Sodium

AKA: Soda crystals

In Ancient Egypt, Egyptians used sodium to create a cleansing agent similar to soap. Using the natural deposits of natron (a mixture consisting mostly of sodium carbonate decahydrate and sodium bicarbonate), Egyptians cleansed and treated the skin.

Later in history, French chemist and surgeon, Nicolas Leblanc, produced sodium carbonate, also known as soda ash, in 1791. Then in 1846, two New York Bankers, John Dwight and Austin Church, established the first factory to develop baking soda from sodium carbonate and carbon dioxide.

Sodium bicarbonate can be used to relieve the itch caused by allergic reactions to plants like poison ivy. As a natural acid neutraliser, it has a soothing and anti-inflammatory effect, preventing further irritation to the skin. Sodium bicarbonate also restores the skin's natural pH balance, leaving it soft and supple.

In homeopathy, several forms of itching may be treated with lotions containing a small portion of carbonate or borate of soda. Alternatively a cup of bi-carb may be added to bath water to soothe

the skin. For chicken pox, a paste made of water and bi-carb may be useful in relieving itching.

10 Uses for Sodium Bicarbonate

1. Laundry sanitiser
2. Deodoriser in sneakers and in bedding for pets; also in cars and on carpets
3. Blends well with vinegar as a household cleanser
4. To make a bath soak
5. Soothe itchy feet
6. Treat insect bites
7. Use as a natural deodorant
8. Facial scrub
9. Use as toothpaste
10. Body exfoliant

Consult your healthcare practitioner.

90. Sophora Flavescens

AKA: Ku shen

S ophora flavescens is a species of plant that comes from the genus or group of organisms known as Sophora. It comes from the large fabaceae family, which includes 52 other species. Nineteen varieties and seven forms of this species are widely distributed in Asia, Oceania and the Pacific islands.

About fifteen species in this genus have a long history of use in traditional Chinese medicine, with the sophora root having multiple variants. Known as Ku Shen in China, this root is commonly used in traditional Chinese medicine.

Both an anti-inflammatory and antioxidant, sophora could possibly be used as a treatment for mast cell-derived allergic inflammatory diseases. Sophora injections have even been known to reduce the toxicity and adverse effects caused by chemotherapy.

Consult your healthcare practitioner.

91. St John's Wort

AKA: Hypericum perforatum

This famous plant has been used as an effective herbal medicine for at least 2400 years. With a medicinal history dating back to Ancient Greece, St John's Wort has been used to treat a variety of ailments. In Ancient Greece, Hippocrates recorded its use for easing hysteria, insomnia, tuberculosis and colds.

The herb supposedly found its name after St John the Baptist, whose birthday occurs when the flowers are in bloom on June 24.

The plant itself is shrubby with clusters of yellow flowers. Both the flowers and leaves are used as medicine. St. John's Wort has been used historically for the topical skin treatment of bruises, mild burns and wounds.

Hyperforin is a constituent of the herb that has been found to have antibacterial activity. One study applied a cream containing St John's Wort to eczema on one side of the body and a placebo cream on the other side for a period of four weeks. The St John's Wort cream showed an improvement in redness, crusting, scaling and skin thickening, together with a reduction of skin infection.

Consult your healthcare practitioner.

92. Sulphur

AKA: *Sulfur/brimstone*

S ulphur is a medicinal agent that has been used for its antiseptic qualities in traditional medicine for over 2,000 years. Extremely popular in Victorian and Edwardian times, sulphur was used as a topical treatment for those suffering from infections, itching and sores.

In modern times, sulphur is used in homeopathy to treat skin diseases such as acne, psoriasis and eczema. Besides reducing itching, sulphur can provide relief from dry, flaky, cracked and reddened skin.

This medicinal agent is prepared from the mineral sulphur. As a homeopathic remedy, pure sulphur powder is watered down with milk or a combination of water and alcohol.

Pure undiluted sulphur has a pungent odour and produces a burning sensation on the skin, much like severe itching. Therefore, the diluted preparation of the mineral makes an ideal homeopathic remedy in the treatment of skin diseases involving itching and burning sensations. In addition to oral preparations, sulphur bath salts, soaps and creams are also available.

But how exactly does sulphur work? Sulphur helps kill off pathogenic microbes on the skin and in the blood. In doing so, it stops damage to the skin tissue and allows the skin to heal.

Researchers have found that Icelanders have low rates of depression, obesity, diabetes, and heart disease, and are attributing much of this to the line of volcanoes that formed the island nation. These volcanoes are full of sulphur ash, which blankets the soil after an eruption and enriches the ground. Drinking water, produce, and meat products contain a dense supply of sulphur.

Consult your healthcare practitioner.

93. Sweet Orange

AKA: Citrus sinensis

Sweet orange trees were brought to Italy, Spain and Portugal from India in the 15ᵗʰ century. Orange trees were then taken to the United States, South America, Africa and Australia.

In some countries, blood oranges are seen as a symbol of the death of Jesus, while in others the fruit is literally fit for a queen. Queen Victoria was once given a coronet of gold and orange blossoms by her husband Albert.

The essential oil of sweet orange is extracted by cold pressing the rinds of the fruit, instilling a fresh and strong aroma. Three oils come from the orange tree. These include orange from the peel, neroli from the flowers and petitgrain from the leaves. Orange oil is a tonic, as well as antiseptic, calmative, anti-inflammatory and diuretic.

Known as a skin tonic, sweet orange oil penetrates deeply into the pores and supports the formation of collagen in the skin. It is great for mature skin, dermatitis, acne and soothing dry irritated skin.

Easy Eczema Salve

You will need:

250g of soft paraffin wax

3 drops of lavender oil

3 drops of chamomile oil

3 drops of sweet orange oil

Method:

1. Combine ingredients in a bowl.
2. Place bowl over a saucepan of hot water.
3. Blend together and let cool slightly.
4. Pour into salve tin for storage.

Calendula oil could replace chamomile oil.

Consult your healthcare practitioner.

94. Tamanu Oil

AKA: Foraha

Although the Tamanu tree is native to East Africa, it is known to grow all over the Southern Hemisphere. Each tree yields just four to five litres of oil per year, which makes this ingredient very expensive. The oil is however, very much worth it. It is believed to have anti-properties that can be used to treat various hair, scalp and skin problems, including eczema.

Tamanu oil possesses a unique capacity to promote the formation of new tissue, thereby accelerating wound healing and the growth of healthy skin. The oil's unusual absorption and luxurious feel, combined with its mild and pleasant aroma, makes it ideal for use in lotions and ointments.

Oil of Tamanu contains three basic classes of lipids (naturally occurring molecules) as well as a unique fatty acid called calophyllum, a novel antibiotic lactone and non-steroidal anti-inflammatory agent called calophyllolide.

Considering that Tamanu is a potent healing agent with proven benefits, it is only a matter of time before Tamanu becomes widely used.

Consult your healthcare practitioner.

95. Turmeric

AKA: Curcuma longa

Turmeric grows wild in the forests of Southern Asia and can be found in Indonesia, India and other nearby Asian countries. Some Pacific islands including Hawaii are also home to this herb.

Turmeric has been widely researched and is found to have many uses. Ideal for healing wounds, turmeric has antioxidant, antiviral, antibacterial, anti-inflammatory and antiseptic properties. While it is used and quoted widely for treating eczema, little data is available to verify this.

Nonetheless, it seems that the active ingredient in turmeric – curcumin – possesses anti-inflammatory and bactericidal properties that may help to treat the inflammation and itching associated with eczema.

Consult your healthcare practitioner.

96. Vitamins

Vitamin A

Vitamin A is a fat-soluble vitamin, meaning it is stored in the body. It is necessary for proper keratinization of the skin. The skin findings associated with vitamin A deficiency are dryness, itching and scaling. Severe deficiency may cause deep skin cracks and fissures.

Vitamin A is found naturally in liver, carrots, eggs, green and yellow vegetables, dairy products and yellow fruits. Consult your healthcare practitioner if you are concerned about a vitamin A deficiency.

Vitamin C

Vitamin C plays a primary role in the formation of collagen, which is important for the growth and repair of body tissue cells, gums, blood vessels, bones and teeth. Collagen is the substance that binds the cells of connective tissue. Vitamin C works as a team with other vitamins, minerals, and enzymes to strengthen the collagen in connective tissue and promote capillary integrity. Vitamin C can also act as an antihistamine.

Vitamin C deficiency (also known as scurvy) can appear as loss of integrity in collagen-containing tissues such as the skin. A symptom of severe scurvy is dry, scaly brown skin.

Vitamin C is found naturally in fresh, raw fruit and vegetables. Alternatively, rose hips are citrus free and hypoallergenic. Consult your healthcare practitioner if you are concerned about a vitamin C deficiency.

Vitamin D

People with eczema have immune systems and skin barriers that don't work properly. Some studies have found that both children and adults with eczema are more likely to have low levels of vitamin D. Research has found that people who have eczema and low levels of vitamin D are more likely to get infections on their skin.

Vitamin D is found naturally in fish oil, fats and dairy products. Consult your healthcare practitioner if you are concerned about a vitamin D deficiency.

Vitamin E

Vitamin E is known for its antioxidant properties, and can help provide relief from itchy skin by improving its texture, keeping it healthy and strong. Vitamin E protects the skin from free radical damage, as well as damage from environmental pollutants.

Vitamin E is found naturally in nuts, vegetable oil, wheat germ, green vegetables and whole grains. Consult your healthcare practitioner if you are concerned about a vitamin E deficiency.

Vitamin K

Vitamin K is typically used to treat blood clotting problems and deficiencies of the vitamin; however some people take vitamin K to alleviate itching associated with biliary cirrhosis, a liver disease. Vitamin K is available in skin creams to treat various conditions.

Vitamin K is found naturally in green leafy vegetable. Consult your healthcare practitioner if you are concerned about a vitamin K deficiency.

Multivitamins usually come in tablet form and are best absorbed when taken after meals and spaced out during the day.

Because some vitamins can be excreted in the urine, taking your vitamins after breakfast, after lunch, and after dinner will give you the highest body level of nutrients. If you must take your vitamins all at once, taking them after the largest meal of the day will usually give the best results.

If you have trouble absorbing nutrients, you may want to consider some of the powdered or liquid vitamins, which don't have to be broken down as much in the gut. Consider taking a children's range of vitamin jubes or pastilles.

97. Walnut Oil

AKA: Juglans regia

Cultivated for over 2000 years, the walnut tree produces a popular, edible nut. While today it is a popular food, in the past walnuts were used in dyes and medicines.

The Chinese and Greeks were the first to cultivate walnuts, followed by the Romans and Europeans. Spreading from country to country, it comes as no surprise that word walnut means 'foreign nut.'

Today the golden brown oil of the walnut is most often used in cooking. Walnut oil is also frequently used in hair and skin preparations and is said to be effective in treating eczema-like conditions. It is an excellent emollient.

Eating just seven walnuts a day may be all it takes to benefit from the antioxidant qualities of the nut. Walnuts can help reduce prostate cancer growth, improve heart health, brainpower and keep weight under control. It is also known improve reproductive health in men.

Walnut Whip Moisturiser

You will need:

½ cup of organic walnut oil

½ cup of organic olive oil

¼ cup of grated beeswax

4 vitamin E capsules

3 drops of geranium oil

3 drops of neroli oil

3 drops of rose oil

Method:

1. Combine ingredients in a bowl.
2. Place bowl over a saucepan of hot water.
3. Stir together and let cool slightly.
4. Blend with a stick blender.
5. Pour into small glass jar.

A combination of these essential oils can be used instead of the above – bergamot, jasmine, clary sage, lavender, petitgrain, sweet orange or sandalwood.

166

Consult your healthcare practitioner.

98. Wheatgerm Oil

AKA: Triticum vulgare

The history of wheat dates back to 7000 BC, with archaeologists finding it in excavations of the world's oldest remains of civilisations.

Wheatgerm oil is extracted by cold pressing. This oil has an amber or brown colour and a pleasant nutty aroma.

Containing high levels of vitamin E, a natural antioxidant that prevents oil from growing rancid quickly, wheatgerm oil is an effective anti-aging tool. In fact, the vitamin E levels of wheatgerm oil are around 3,500 p*arts per million (ppm)* compared to 250-600 ppm in other plant-based oils. These natural antioxidants help wheatgerm soften the skin and boost cell regeneration. For this reason, wheatgerm is a suitable treatment for dry itchy skin.

You can include wheatgerm in your diet by adding it to breakfast cereals, casseroles, milk or pancakes.

Wheatgerm and Oat Pancakes

You will need:

2 eggs, lightly beaten

2 cups of milk

2 teaspoons of sodium bicarbonate

8 tablespoons of wheatgerm

1/2 cup of finely ground oats

100g of self-raising flour

Oil for cooking

Method:

1. Blend all the ingredients together in a medium size bowl.
2. Pour a tablespoon of mixture in a frying pan.
3. Cook until bubbles appear on the top.
4. Flip lightly and cook for 2 minutes.
5. Remove from heat and fill with your favourite topping.

Consult your healthcare practitioner.

99. Witch Hazel

AKA: *Hamamelis virginiana*

This plant extract was widely used for medicinal purposes by American Indians, who boiled the plant and used the extract, known as 'magic water,' to treat swellings, inflammations and tumours. Early Puritan settlers in New England adopted this remedy from the natives. Since then its use has become widely established throughout the United States.

The word 'witch' in the name of this herb is actually derived from the Anglo-Saxon word *wych,* meaning flexible. Indeed, witch hazel lives up to its name, proving to be effective tool for treating the many symptoms of eczema.

Witch hazel is known to relieve itching and help with 'weeping' or oozing eczema. In one study, 22 patients with eczema were treated with a standardised witch hazel salve on one arm and a non-steroidal anti-inflammatory cream on the other, over the course of three weeks. While the non-steroidal anti-inflammatory cream worked, the witch hazel was just as effective for reducing the redness, scaling, and itching.

Consult your healthcare practitioner.

100. Yellow Dock

AKA: Rumex crispus

A well-known traditional medicine, yellow dock has been used as a medicinal plant since ancient times. A favourite among old time doctors, settlers and herbal practitioners, yellow dock continues to be used today and has a particularly rich history in North America. Native Americans frequently used the plant as an external remedy for skin ailments.

The tannin or micronutrient content is responsible for the astringent effect of yellow dock, making it effective in relieving various skin conditions when used internally.

An ointment of yellow dock is also valuable for eruptive skin conditions that cause itching, sores, and scabby lesions. When applied topically in ointments and poultices, yellow dock relieves itchy skin, scabies, ringworm and eczema.

Consult your healthcare practitioner.

101. Zinc Oxide

AKA: ZnO

During the 1st century, Greek physician Dioscorides discussed the use of a zinc oxide ointment in his work. Zinc oxide is also talked of in the ancient medical encyclopaedia, *The Canon of Medicine,* written by Persian polymath Avicenna in 1025 AD. Here it is described as Avicenna's preferred treatment for a variety of skin conditions, including cancer.

Today zinc oxide is combined with around 0.5 per cent iron oxide to make the popular calamine lotion. Zinc oxide is also used in a variety of other products such as anti-dandruff shampoo and antiseptic, as well as baby powder and creams. It can be used to treat a wide range of skin conditions including eczema, nappy rash and more.

Despite the wide range of topical treatments on the market, working from the inside to maintain your skin's natural protective coating is just as important. It is also important to note that zinc deficiency itself can cause dry skin with a rough, scaly appearance.

Natural Sources of Zinc

Oysters

Fish

Liver

Brewer's yeast

Eggs

Whole grains

Pumpkin seeds

Mushrooms

Consult your healthcare practitioner.

Index of Remedies**

A

Acupuncture 15

Almond Oil 17

Aloe Vera 18

Antimony 20

Apple Cider Vinegar 21

Apricot Kernel Oil 23

Arsenic 24

B

Benzoin 26

Bergamot 28

Birch 30

Bismuth 32

Bleach Baths 33

Borage Seed Oil 34

Bromelain 35

Burdock 36

C

Calendula 38

Camphor 40

Carrot Oil 42

Cedarwood 44

Chamomile Oil 45

Chickweed 46

Cleavers 48

Coal Tar 49

Coconut Oil 50

Comfrey 52

Cumin Seed Oil 53

Cypress 54

D

Diet 56

E

Echinacea 58

Elderberry 60

Environment 62

Eucalyptus 65

Evening Primrose Oil 67

F

Fish Oil 69

Flavonoids 70

Frankincense 71

Fumitory 73

G

Geranium 75

Goat Milk 77

Goldenseal 79

Gotu Kola 81

H

Heartsease 83

Hemp Seed Oil 84

Homeopathy 85

Horsetail 87

Hydrocortisione 88

Hypnotherapy 90

I

Immunosuppressants 92

** Information on the remedies described in this book is for educational use only and not intended as medical advice. Remedies in this book may trigger side effects and interfere with other medications, herbs and supplements. Please consult your healthcare practitioner (herbalist, naturopath, homeopath or general practitioner) before self-administering a herb or remedy.

Iron 93

J
Jewelweed–Pale and Spotted 94
Jojoba Oil 97
Juniper 98

K
Kukui Nut Oil 100
Kunzea 101

L
Lavender 102
Liquorice 104

M
Magnesium 106
Marshmallow 108
Milk Thistle 109
Minerals 111
Mugwort 112
Myrrh 113

N
Neem 115

O
Oats 116
Opiates 118
Oregon Grape Root 119

P
Parsley 120
Patchouli 121
Pawpaw 123
Peach Kernel Oil 124
Perilla Seed Oil 125
Phosphorus 126
Plantain 128
Probiotics 130
Purslane 131

R
Red Clover 132
Rice Bran 134
Rosehip Oil 135
Rosemary 137
Rosewood 139

S
Safflower Oil 140
Salicylic Acid 141
Salt 142

Sandalwood 144
Sarsaparilla 146
Sea Buckthorn 148
Silver 149
Slippery Elm 151
Sodium 152
Sophora Flavescens 154
St John's Wort 155
Sulphur 156
Sweet Orange 158

T
Tamanu Oil 160
Turmeric 161

V
Vitamins 162

W
Walnut Oil 165
Wheatgerm Oil 167
Witch Hazel 169

Y
Yellow Dock 170

Z
Zinc Oxide 171

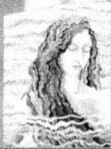

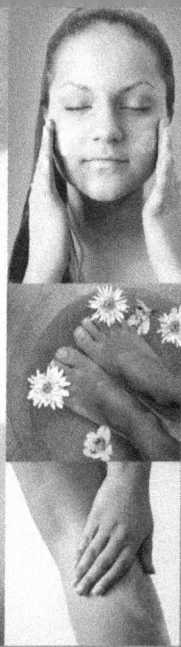

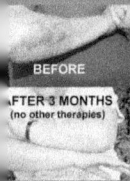

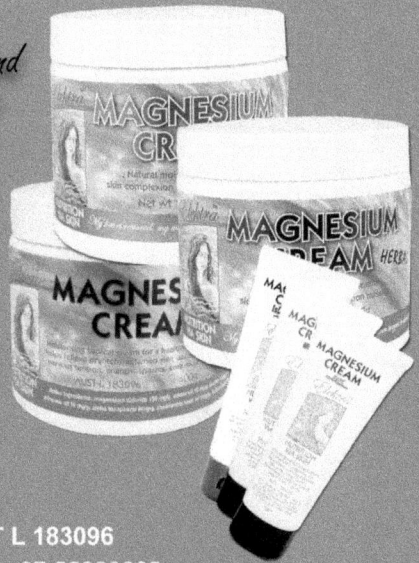

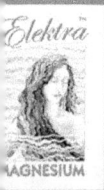

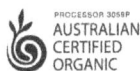

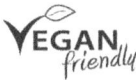

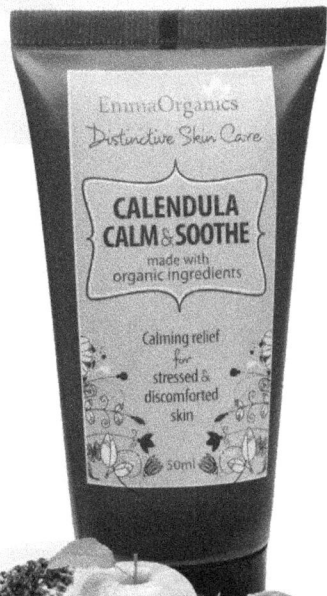

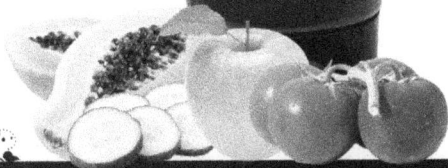

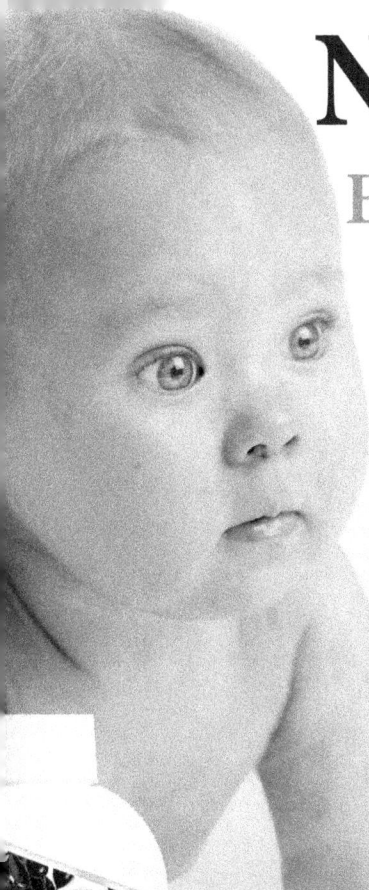
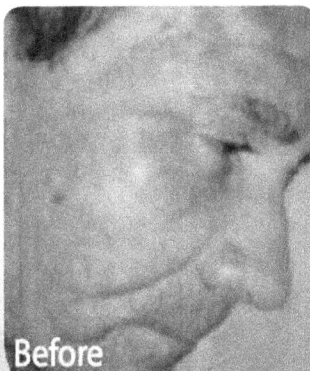
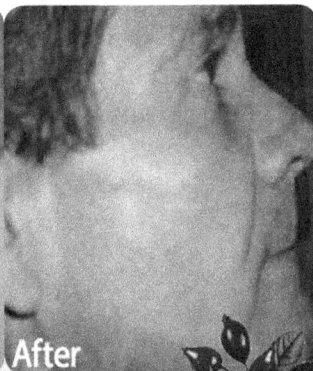
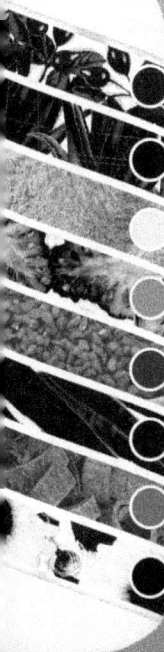
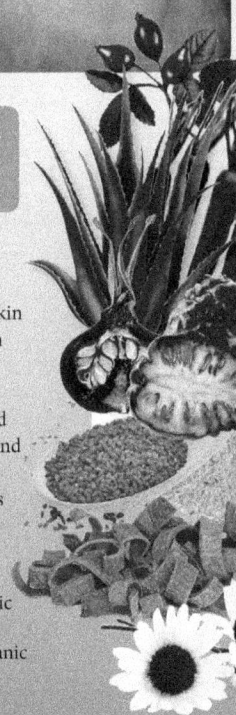
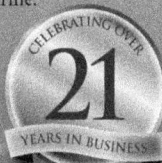
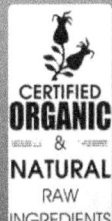

DRY, FLAKY, ITCHY SKIN?

Maximum hydration for todays travellers

- ✓ SPECIFICALLY FORMULATED FOR AIRLINE PASSENGERS AND CABIN CREW TO MAINTAIN OPTIMAL SKIN HYDRATION
- ✓ 16 CERTIFIED ORGANIC INGREDIENTS
- ✓ A MULTI-ACTIVE MOISTURISER CONTAINING ANTI-OXIDANTS, NUT, SEED AND PLANT EXTRACTS AND OILS
- ✓ SOFTENS, HYDRATES AND MOISTURISES DURING AIR TRAVEL
- ✓ IDEAL FOR FACE AND HANDS – WHEREVER SKIN IS EXPOSED TO LOW HUMIDITY
- ✓ HANDY TRAVEL PURSE OR POCKET SIZE

SHOP ONLINE

aviationhydration.com.au

facebook.com /aviationhydration

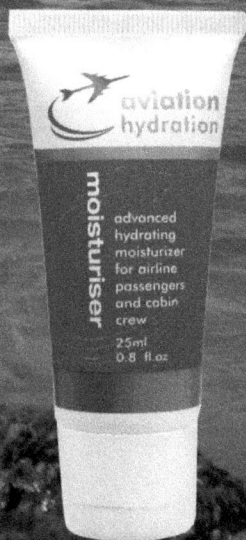

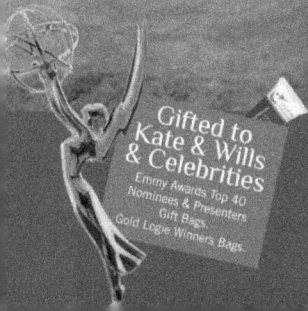

aviation hydration

moisturiser

advanced hydrating moisturizer for airline passengers and cabin crew

25ml 0.8 fl.oz

Gifted to Kate & Wills & Celebrities
Emmy Awards Top 40 Nominees & Presenters Gift Bags.
Gold Logie Winners Bags.

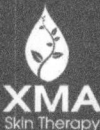

XMA Skin Therapy

Aviation Hydration
The perfect travel partner

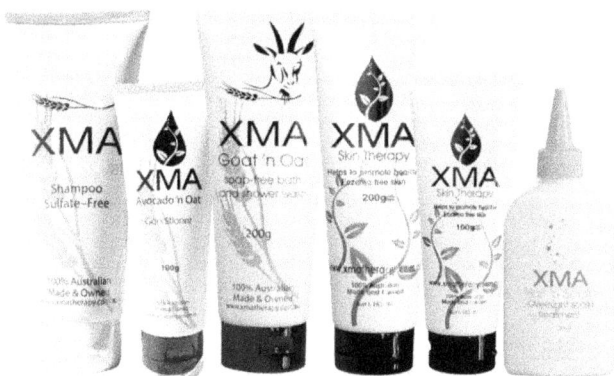

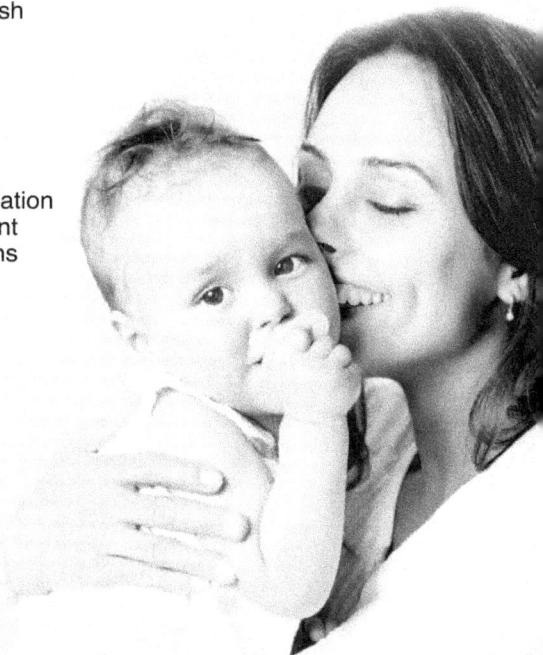

eaa

eczema association australasia
support education management

www.eczema.org.au
1300 300 182
help@eczema.org.au

MEMBERSHIP
(Annual Family Membership Fee $39)

Benefits of Membership:

- Quarterly Magazine with tips, articles, recipes and details of latest products
- Access to the member only area on our website
- Free samples of products
- Social Register (optional) - you can get in touch with people in your area and for example, arrange a coffee morning
- Information sheets covering a wide range of topics
- We have access to Health Professionals for help and information on the latest treatments

MEMBERSHIP APPLICATION FORM

☐ Social Register
☐ Media Availability

Sufferer's Name

Applicant's Name

Address

Postcode

Telephone

Email

I enclose my cheque payable to the
ECZEMA ASSOCIATION OF AUSTRALASIA INC
PO Box 1784 DC CLEVELAND QLD 4163

Or please charge my ☐ Mastercard ☐ Visa ☐ American Express

Card Number

☐☐☐☐ ☐☐☐☐ ☐☐☐☐ ☐☐☐☐

Expiry Date

Card Check Value   (last 3 numbers on back of card)   ☐☐☐

Card Name

Signature

PRIVACY ACT: Membership information collected is stored on our electronic database, which is password protected, and in our lockable filing cabinet. No information is distributed to a third party without your express permission, eg for our social register, and with the exception of any information as required by our professional advisers such as solicitors, accountants and auditors.

The Eczema Association of Australasia Inc supports and educates Eczema sufferers and carers, along with the wider community, in all aspects of Eczema and its impact.

www.ingramcontent.com/pod-product-compliance
Lightning Source LLC
Chambersburg PA
CBHW072132020426
42334CB00018B/1770